ASSISTED
SUICIDE

ASSISTED

THEORY AND PRACTICE IN ELECTIVE DEATH

SUICIDE

C. G. PRADO & S. J. TAYLOR

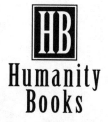

Humanity
Books

an imprint of Prometheus Books
59 John Glenn Drive, Amherst, New York 14228-2197

Published 1999 by Humanity Books, an imprint of Prometheus Books

03 02 01 00 99   5 4 3 2 1

Library of Congress Cataloging-in-Publication Data

Prado, C. G.
    Assisted suicide : theory and practice in elective death / C.G. Prado and S.J. Taylor.
        p.   cm.
    Includes bibliographical references and index.
    ISBN 1–57392–634–5 (alk. paper). — ISBN 1–57392–633–7 (pbk. : alk. paper)
    1. Assisted suicide—Moral and ethical aspects. 2. Euthanasia—Moral and
ethical aspects. 3. Taylor, S. J., 1941–   . II. Title.
R726.P73   1999
174'.24—DC21   98–15513
                                                                    CIP

Printed in the United States of America on acid-free paper

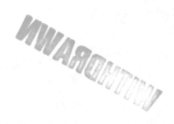

For Catherine.
C.G.P.

For Don.
S.J.T.

"When my time comes, I hope my doctor will have read this book. . . . [It] is indispensable for anyone—legislators, doctors, patients' relatives, patients themselves—trying conscientiously to make principled decisions as to when the prolongation of life is in patients' interest, and when it is not. In stressing the overriding importance of respect for patients' autonomy it is an effective counter to threatened bureaucratization of dying."

—Wallace Matson
Professor of Philosophy, Emeritus
University of California, Berkeley

"[This book] achieves two remarkable feats: it cuts to the heart of the theoretical issues while keeping a resolutely clear view of the practical dilemmas. . . . [Its] striking originality, among the many discussions of physician-assisted suicide now on the market, lies in its taking epistemological and not just ethical questions about suicide as central."

—Margaret P. Battin
Professor, Philosophy Department
University of Utah

Free to die and free in death,
able to say a holy No
when the time for Yes has passed.

Friedrich Nietzsche, *Thus Spake Zarathustra*

CONTENTS

PREFACE

Our aim in writing this book is to contribute to the ethical guidance that is becoming so necessary regarding assisted suicide. Despite its present illegality, and Dr. Jack Kevorkian's recent murder conviction in Michigan, assistance in suicide is currently being provided under various guises, a practice that will continue. It is also likely that some form of assisted suicide soon will be, if not legalized, then widely condoned on a more open basis than at present. These developments are being forced by a climate in which the abandonment of life in calamitous circumstances is increasingly seen as justified, notwithstanding moral, religious, and legal prohibitions.

Present provision of assistance in suicide or voluntary euthanasia turns on how most physicians distinguish between *killing* and *letting die* with respect to the discontinuance of "aggressive" life-sustaining treatment in terminal cases. The distinction is made between actually causing death and allowing underlying pathological causes to result in death. But closer examination often shows that "letting die" really is *helping* to die, and that the difference between "active" and "passive" involvement in patients' deaths is very unclear and diversely interpreted. As a result, guidance is urgently needed if caregivers willing to hasten otherwise hard deaths are to do so in the most responsible and justified ways possible.

The heart of our contribution to this necessary guidance is a set of criteria for assessing the rationality of suicide and so of assistance in its commission.[1] But it is how we consider the criteria that makes this book special. The key point is that, although we agree on the criteria, we differ on their implementation. One of us, confident of philosophical and moral theory's efficacy, believes that the criteria define permissible suicide and assisted suicide and require strict application. The other, familiar with the vagaries of clinical practice, believes that the criteria can serve only as guidelines and require contextual interpretation. We both think there are ways to determine when it's right to end one's own life or to help suffering individuals end their lives rather than endure the torment of terminal illness. However, one of us believes that abstractions can only guide caregivers' participation in elective death and that empathic understanding of particular predicaments is what mainly legitimizes that participation. The other believes that a caregiver's participation must conform to a universal, and thus necessarily abstract, demarcation of allowable acts and that empathic considerations cannot play a decisive role. The consequence is that, in the very working out and considering of the criteria, we illustrate and address the tensions between theory and practice.

The differences between us reflect a basic division in widely held attitudes toward assisted suicide. Though a growing number of professionals and nonprofessionals concerned with assisted suicide acknowledge that it is advisable and permissible in exceptional cases, many balk at accepting assistance in suicide as a sanctioned practice. They believe, as one of us does, that permissibility of assisted suicide is governed by precepts and fear that legalization will encourage us to grow too lenient in the application of those precepts. Others see no point in acknowledging occasional permissibility if assisted suicide must remain covert and officially criminal. They believe, as the other of us does, that the very empathy that legitimizes assistance in suicide is a better guard against abuse than illegality; they also fear that protective legislation will cause many to endure agonizing days and months they'd sooner forgo.

Our goal and hope is that what follows will not only provide caregivers with a sound basis for making some tough decisions, but that the tensions evident in our differing inclinations to favor contextual interpretation or strict application of the criteria will alert caregivers and concerned others to the complexities of those decisions.

NOTE

1. The criteria were initially worked out in Prado 1990.

I

THEORY AND PRACTICE

Court cases in the United States and Canada, and attendant media coverage, have transformed assisted suicide from an unspoken practice to a pressing social issue.[1] Assisted suicide has joined abortion as one of the major and most intractable issues of our time, and recent developments indicate that despite setbacks,[2] an aging population and resultant changes in social values will foster wider acceptance of assisted suicide and its eventual legalization.[3] Despite the Supreme Court's recent upholding of New York and Washington states' lower-court bans on assisted suicide, on the grounds that assisted suicide isn't "a fundamental liberty interest protected by the due-process clause,"[4] the ruling wasn't preclusive and leaves the issue to individual states.[5] But contrary to the impression conveyed by current media coverage, legalization is actually not the central issue regarding assisted suicide. It isn't as if we were in the midst of a public debate about whether or not to allow assisted suicide. The debate is about sanctioning a current, albeit limited practice; the debate is about removing criminal prohibitions, not about initiating a practice.[6] Assisted suicide is practiced *now*, regardless of its illegality.[7] This is especially true with respect to certain groups of patients who face drawn-out and terribly punishing deaths.[8] Whether unspoken or described as cessation of treatment, assisted suicide is being done.[9] "What might be called managed deaths . . . are now the norm in the United States."[10] The truly important questions are about whether suicide ever *makes good sense*, whether *assisting* suicide is ever permissible, and if so, what professional ethics should govern its provision.[11]

13

Like abortion, assisted suicide raises profound questions that pose moral, social, and political dilemmas. As with abortion, the dilemmas will continue unresolved because they arise from a clash of profoundly divergent conceptions of personal autonomy and the nature of human life. Whether it's the life of a fetus or of an eighty-year-old, the basic split is between those who emphasize autonomy and believe that life is the possession of the person who lives it,[12] and those who emphasize responsibility and "view life as a gift, of which we are custodians with certain duties."[13] This isn't a difference likely to be overcome by argument, and with both abortion and assisted suicide, the most we can hope for are reasonable compromises. But also like abortion, assisted suicide is practiced regardless of legality. It is this hard fact that makes questions about governing ethics exigent ones.

Aside from spouses and partners who help their companions to die,[14] some physicians and nurses[15] are openly assisting the commission of suicide.[16] They are challenging existing law as others did two decades ago by performing abortions.[17] But for every media-covered case of assisted suicide, there are hundreds that go unremarked. For every clinician intent on publicly testing suicide's illegality, there are many who quietly help patients to die who want to avoid unnecessary agony in terminal illness.[18] This is most commonly done in hospital settings under the guise of refusal and requested cessation of life-supporting treatment. People do commit "surcease" suicide or suicide in intolerable and hopeless situations; often they need help in doing so, and despite legal prohibitions, they are increasingly getting that help when they request it.[19]

It is important, though, that when aid in dying is provided, it is sometimes unclear whether that aid is best described as assistance in the commission of *suicide* or as provision of voluntary euthanasia.[20] The importance of the distinction has to do with what ethical and legal factors govern or prohibit the actions of someone rendering assistance. Unfortunately, the fact is that assisted suicide is a more acceptable idea to many than is euthanasia, because in suicide, the responsibility for the act is the agent's own. In euthanasia, someone else bears the primary responsibility for the death of the person helped to die. Instances of voluntary euthanasia are therefore sometimes redescribed as assisted suicide for various purposes.[21] If our society is going to accept the practice of assisted suicide, it must face the question of whether it will also accept the practice of some forms of euthanasia. But our main concern is with *assisted suicide*. However difficult the distinction between it and voluntary euthanasia may be to maintain in actual cases, our concern with voluntary euthanasia is secondary, and what we say about assisted suicide applies to voluntary euthanasia only by implication and extension. The significance of this focus has to do with the primacy we give to the autonomy of self-destructive decisions.

THE PROJECT

There are good, humane reasons to provide assistance in suicide both in terminal situations and when chronic conditions prove unendurable.[22] Suicide may be the most sensible choice for a person when sound reasoning determines that self-destruction is what best serves that person's interests and values. When that is the case, incapacity to commit suicide unaided shouldn't prevent people from doing what is best for them. Others who are willing to lend assistance in the commission of suicide should be able to do so without incurring criminal penalties, so assisted suicide should be legalized if we can work out ways to curb possible abuse.

But because assisted suicide is in fact being provided by clinicians under a variety of descriptions, it is imperative that ethics to govern its permissibility be provided even though the legal issue is still unresolved.[23] Society can't wait for the legalization of assisted suicide to offer ethical guidance to those entrusted with the care of the terminally ill, the very old, and the severely impaired, who engage in it with some claim to legitimacy. We must insure that when assistance in suicide is provided, it is permissible and proper. Those clinicians who stretch, circumvent, or defy existing laws by assisting the commission of suicide are, in effect, making policy regarding the practice. In a democratic society, courts and governments ultimately follow when legislative prohibitions are successfully challenged, so those who pose the challenges largely determine the nature of the practices that are legalized. It could prove disastrous if we allow ethically problematic practices to develop and then enshrine those practices in statutes if we legalize assisted suicide.

The irony is that effective ethical guidance for assisted suicide is not lacking for want of effort; it is lacking because of conflict and dissent. The fundamentality of the split, between seeing life as a disposable possession and seeing it as an unrenounceable gift, means that ethical theory about assisted suicide is as divided as are practical and legal views. The immediate consequence is that those looking for ethical guidance regarding assisted suicide tend to read and listen to those theorists with whom they basically agree for more general reasons, such as moral or religious persuasion. Despite the fact that this tendency is likely counterproductive, it is understandable, because when one looks for help with serious questions, one naturally turns to those one respects and trusts.[24]

There are other reasons for the gap between ethical theory and clinical practice. The most obvious is clinicians' reservations about ethical theoreticians' grasp of the concrete realities of day-to-day practice. Clinicians tend to see their own practical decisions as commonsensical and as dictated by the immediate well-being of their patients. They find it hard to think that anyone not actively engaged with patients could have the incentive or opportunity to truly understand, much less resolve, issues about what is or isn't permissible when someone sorely afflicted chooses not to live under those conditions. Clinicians are understandably impatient with theoretical ideas that seem too distant from actual cases to bear on their activities. When clinicians seek ethical guidance in their work, they turn to discussion of case studies.[25] The underlying assumption is that there is more to be learned from accounts of case histories and judgment calls related by experienced clinicians[26] than from abstract treatises and presentations.[27] Unfortunately, theoreticians do tend to assume too readily that they understand the clinical contexts in which their abstractions are realized. They underestimate the impact of day-to-day experience on clinicians' attitudes and underrate clinicians' need to take decisive action in urgent and often emotionally fraught situations. For their part, clinicians are often too impatient with the need to draw sometimes subtle distinctions and to be precise with terminology.[28]

The result is a surface impression that ethical theoreticians and practicing clinicians are engaged in separate activities having little to do with each other. The gap between theory and practice is further widened by adoption of unproductive attitudes: Clinicians become dismissive of theory, and theoreticians become condescending toward practice. These attitudes are reinforced by a lack of corrective communication, a lack caused by clinicians' shortage of time to read and digest lengthy theoretical treatments of medical issues and theoreticians' inability to summarize complex arguments without vitiating their own efforts at thorough analysis.

Still, the most serious and apparently intractable reason for the gap between theory and practice is the one noted earlier: Theoretical work on assisted suicide is inevitably shaped by theoreticians' own moral and religious commitments. This means that all too often, instead of providing a basis for the resolution of practical disputes about the permissibility of assisted suicide, theoreticians only reproduce those disputes in conflicting theories.[29] For their part, clinicians avail themselves of those theories that best suit their own views and practices. In this way, assisted suicide again shows remarkable parallels with abortion. Those who theorize about abortion are usually committed to one or another moral, religious, or political position, and their pro or con arguments are invariably more often reiterations of their commitments than impartial attempts to resolve hard issues. In both cases, clinicians are left with a partisan diversity that, like many sermons, offers guidance only to the converted.

The fundamental split on the nature and value of human life means that the gap between ethical theory and clinical practice is deeper than unproductive attitudes. But even more profound than diversity of underlying moral and religious commitments is another reason for the gap, one that explains why clinicians regularly find themselves unable to effectively apply even their own theoretical principles in particular cases. The difficult truth of the matter is that irresolvable conflicts arise between ethical theory and clinical practice regarding assisted suicide. The demands of the theoretical and the practical regarding the permissibility of assisted suicide are often irreconcilable. The expectation that enough work could produce consistent theory-based and readily applicable rules for dealing with assisted suicide is a barren one. The relation of ethical theory to the clinical practice it supposedly governs is unlike that of scientific theory's productive relation to technology.[30] When the issue is whether or not to help someone take their[31] own life, theory and practice usually clash because they make contrary demands on clinicians.[32] Ethical theory requires that clinicians adhere to general principles in deciding what to do about requests for assisted suicide. But good medical practice requires that they accommodate particular circumstances in making their decisions.[33] This clash of requirements is why principles sometimes look inapplicable or irrelevant, and why decisions about assisted suicide must always be compromises between the conflicting demands of theory-generated principles and practical exigencies.

The upshot of the foregoing difficulties is that while ethical theoreticians manufacture unproductive theories having only marginal influence on clinicians who share the anguish of protracted death, clinicians establish practices that range from the merely idiosyncratic to the dangerously misconceived. But the gap between theory and practice can't and needn't be accepted as a hopeless impasse. Once we understand the nature of the more serious conflicts between theory and practice, we will appreciate that although the theory-practice gap can't be closed, it can be bridged. Many of the conflicts between theoretical principles and clinical practices call not for resolution but for compromise. What must be striven for is a *balance* of theoretical and practical considerations in making clinical decisions about assisted suicide. Striving for balanced compromise is our only realistic option with respect to bridging the theory-practice gap, and the gap must be bridged. Without theoretical principles to establish consistency and determine priorities, clinicians may be tyrannized by their personal responses; without practical accommodation to varying contextual realities, they may blunt their compassion and neglect desperate need. For their part, without appreciation of the practical application of their work, theoreticians will engage only one another in arcane and practically unproductive debate.

The aim of this book is to help facilitate a balancing of the conflicting demands of theory and practice regarding assisted suicide. Our strategy is to explore the implications of three minimal theoretical requirements, in order to bring out what may be most basically at odds in the perspectives of ethical theoreticians and clinicians regarding assisted suicide. We accept in principle the moral permissibility of both suicide and assisted suicide. Our interest is in the question of the *rationality* of suicide and assisted suicide. As we argue, the question of the rationality of suicide is logically prior to the question of its morality, since only rational acts can be morally culpable. We address only the prior question, and our objective is to enable compromise on decisions about the provision of assisted suicide by clarifying what is most fundamentally at issue when minimal theoretical requirements conflict with practical demands. We proceed by providing a basic set of three criteria for assessing the rationality of suicide and thus the permissibility of assisted suicide.[34]

Our criteria set out what we agree are axiomatic conditions for suicide to be a rational choice for someone. We also agree that only if the criteria are satisfied—i.e., only if suicide is a rational option—is it ethically and morally[35] permissible to assist in its commission. But the criteria provide only the basic structure for our project. What makes this book special is how we proceed in light of our *dis*agreement about how the criteria establish when suicide is rational enough to warrant assistance in its commission.

The key point is that while we agree that the criteria demonstrate that suicide can be rational, we disagree on both their status and their implementation. The disagreement is rooted in how our similar training has been differently applied in our day-to-day work. One of us spends his working time pondering epistemological questions, and the other spends her working time forging ethical answers. One of us is confident of theory's ability to produce reliable and universalizable principles to govern assisted suicide. Therefore, the main task seems to be the establishment of criteria for rational suicide and permissible assisted suicide on the basis of abstract considerations. Given their conceptual nature, once those criteria are established, they require strict application. The other of us is intimately familiar with the complexities of concrete situations and confident of the wisdom of pragmatic and caring clinical decisions. Therefore, the main task seems to be the derivation of criteria from practices that are productive not because they conform to abstract principles but because they yield consistently good results. The criteria follow on good practice and serve not as determinants but as guides, so they always need contextual interpretation.

Precisely because our respective approaches are theory-based and -oriented and practice-based and -oriented, our collaboration results in constructive exploration of those situations in which conflicts arise between the demands of theory and of practice. We are able to jointly consider issues in a more informed way than a single approach would allow, and we present those issues in a manner that will engage both theoreticians and clinicians. We think that in the process of reading the results of our combined—sometimes coincident, sometimes contrary—views on assisted suicide, theoretically inclined readers will benefit from seeing familiar abstract requirements for permissible assisted suicide contrasted with less familiar practical demands, and practically inclined readers will benefit from seeing how those familiar practical demands relate to less familiar abstract requirements. We hope that clinicians will better appreciate that the gap they see between their practices and ethical theory is caused not by the failings of theory or theorists but by how application of the general to the particular is always an exacting but inherently conditional process.[36] We also hope that theoreticians will better appreciate the complex texture of the practical situations in which their work is applied and how absolute principles must sometimes be qualified to productively govern what people actually do.

MAKING A START

The pivotal question raised by the conflicting requirements and demands of ethical theory and clinical practice is whether abstract principles or the messy contours of actual cases should take precedence in shaping decisions about assisted suicide. The question is one of priorities: In the making of decisions about assisting willful self-destruction, what should come first and most directly govern the permissibility of assisted suicide, theoretical abstractions or concrete realities? This question should not be misconstrued as a choice between caricatures of legalistic rigidity and easy accommodation. The question is the ancient and difficult one of how best to achieve reasonable adherence to principles that can't be applied exactly and unequivocally to the actual cases they are supposed to govern.[37]

It may initially look, particularly to philosophers, as if the priority question is really the choice between traditionally opposed deontological and consequentialist moral theories. This is because deontological or duty-based morality gives priority to principles, whereas consequentialist or result-determined morality, most notably utilitarianism, considers moral principles defeasible guides or rules of thumb and gives priority to the effects of action. But contemporary professional ethics, especially medical ethics, draws from both deontological and consequentialist sources, despite their traditional exclusivity.[38] In particular, professional ethics takes the principle of autonomy (respect for persons' free choices) from deontology and the principles of nonmaleficence ("do no harm") and beneficence ("bring about good") from consequentialism or utilitarianism. The answer to the priority question can't be found in one or the other moral theory or even in an eclectic collection of principles, because the question is about the application of principles, and no theory, much less individual principles, can contain exhaustive directions for their own application.

One of us thinks that what needs to be added to application of theory-generated principles in determining the permissibility of assisted suicide is empathy in the assessment of requests for assisted suicide. Empathy may warrant qualification of the deontological autonomy principle and govern interpretation of the consequentialist beneficence principle. *Empathy*, as used here, draws on the ordinary sense of sensitive compassion, but it also has the technical sense of "emotional knowing of another human being rather than intellectual understanding" of a person's circumstances.[39] The key idea is that empathy complements the traditional ethical perspective of the detached observer with that of the empathic participant in the making of clinical decisions about the permissibility of assisted suicide. Seeing empathy as having a decisive role in determining the permissibility of assisted suicide results from believing that abstract principles can only guide a clinician's participation in assisted suicide, and that it is empathic understanding of particular predicaments that legitimizes that participation. In this view, clinicians should adopt the perspective of the empathic participant and take up that of the detached observer only as a check on their involvement.

Here, ethics is "a mode of thinking that is contextual and narrative rather than formal and abstract."[40] This means that governing ethical principles are defeasible guides, and the role of empathy is constitutive rather than ameliorative, because it determines what counts as an applicable principle. Principles are defeasible because they are not prior determinants of permissible practice but recapitulations of practices that have been judged productive.

While we agree that empathy figures importantly in decisions about whether assisted suicide is permissible, we differ on whether the technical sense of empathy is viable, and thus on how decisive a role empathy can play. The other of us believes that a clinician's participation in assisted suicide should conform to universal principles that determine the permissibility of assisted suicide, so clinicians should adopt the perspective of the detached observer and permit empathic understanding only a tempering role. The reason is that, in this opposing view, ethics is essentially formal, and ethical principles governing assisted suicide are unconditional, so the role of empathy is secondary; empathy may qualify the application of a principle only when the principle allows it or is ambiguous.

The criteria provided in the next chapter derive from the principles of autonomy, nonmaleficence, and beneficence and enable the making of sound decisions about when suicide is for the best and thus when it is permissible to help someone else commit suicide who cannot do so unaided.[41] The criteria are, in the first instance, for rational[42] *un*assisted suicide, because the primary need is to establish that choosing to end one's own life can be rational in the sense of being the best means to achieve the best purpose. This requires that the process of deciding to commit suicide conform to established principles of reason, that suicide be in the individual's best interests, and that suicide be in accord with the individual's values. For suicide to be the best means to the best purpose, it must also be in accordance with the individual's obligations to others. However, those obligations vary so much from case to case that they can only be acknowledged here, and we subsume them under reference to values.[43]

By *rational suicide*, we mean suicide that is the best means to achieve the best purpose, where "the best means" is the action that sound reasoning determines is optimal to most effectively achieve a given objective in a particular situation, and where "the best purpose" is the objective that is most beneficial to the agent's interests and values.

Provision of credible criteria for rational suicide is intended to show the wrongness of the prevalent but mistaken view that suicide is irrational. Many believe that choosing to die is always aberrant, that it is "against nature" for an individual to willingly give up life,[44] that "suicide is generally and correctly assumed to be the expression of a pathological state of mind, usually depression."[45] If suicide were always irrational, assisted suicide would never be permissible, because such assistance would always compound a wrong by contributing to an irrational destructive act. But as the criteria show, there are specifiable conditions that, when met, make suicide rational.

It is also a common and mistaken view that choosing to die is always wrong because it is morally prohibited. This view is mistaken because suicide could always be wrong only if it contravened a universal moral principle, and moral codes differ on this point. Not only do some moral codes tolerate suicide, but there are those that hold it to be an honorable act of atonement.[46] Lacking universal prohibition, suicide may be permissible despite particular moral prohibitions. If an individual's moral code does forbid suicide, however rational it may be, that person may choose to respect the prohibition.[47] However, it is possible for a person to abandon or contravene a moral code that prohibits suicide and to do so for good reason, for instance, if the prohibition of suicide is judged to be inadequately justified or based only on some form of paternalism.

Just as someone may opt to respect a moral code's prohibition of suicide, someone may simply choose not to commit suicide despite its being rational to do so. Even if it is rational to end one's life, that isn't by itself a conclusive reason to commit suicide. Philosopher David Hume would remind us that reason should only serve our wants and needs.[48] In a situation in which suicide is the best course of action, a person may choose to live on, perhaps gambling that things might improve. It is even clearer that the rationality of one individual's suicide can't compel another individual to participate in its commission. Someone asked to assist suicide might not want to assume any responsibility for another's death.

Once it is shown that it can be rational and not necessarily immoral to commit suicide, it is possible to justify assisted suicide as both rational and moral. Showing assisted suicide to be a rational choice is largely a matter of establishing that if suicide is the best means to achieve the best purpose for one individual, but that individual can't commit suicide without help, the rationality of the act invites the willing participation of another individual who recognizes the rationality of the act. Rationality is common to all,[49] so one individual's sound reasoning should have the same force for another. But this remains a matter of invitation, not obligation; the person concerned is free to not assist, and there is the moral dimension to consider. Showing assisted suicide to be moral is a different matter, because the deciding factor is not the rationality of the first individual's act but the moral principles governing the second individual's conduct. Given that suicide is the best course of action for one person does not automatically decide the moral question for another person about assisting its commission. Unlike common rationality, the moral codes of the two people may differ.[50] When the rationality criteria are satisfied and there is a genuine desire to die but an inability to commit suicide unaided, it is neither rationality nor moral obligation but compassion that makes someone act as an extension of another's will and need.[51]

Aside from the questions of suicide's rationality and morality, another major obstacle to acceptance of assisted suicide as a justifiable practice is the widespread but problematic belief that once assisted suicide is legalized or even tacitly condoned, it will be systematically abused. Though a growing number of concerned people acknowledge that assisted suicide is permissible in exceptional cases, many balk at accepting it as a sanctioned practice.[52] Their fear is that social acceptance and/or legalization of assisted suicide will encourage dangerous permissiveness and eventual laxity in its use. They worry that assisted suicide won't be "the option of last resort" but rather "the attractive solution of first resort."[53]

The standard articulation of the view that assisted suicide is too dangerous to condone, much less legalize, is the "slippery slope" argument.[54] The argument is used against acceptance or legalization of euthanasia as well as of assisted suicide, and it is used both by those who acknowledge the rare permissibility of assisted suicide and by those who oppose it categorically. The slippery slope argument is that societal acceptance of assisted suicide will inevitably invite abuse and lead to arbitrary medical murder. Even granting the best intentions, opponents of assisted suicide feel that because of its inherent wrongness, assisted suicide, like abortion, will be done in defiance of natural inclination, and its practice will turn "into a kind of compulsion, as if the more times [practitioners] do it, the more they are assured it is right."[55] The reasoning, then, is that although assisted suicide may be permissible in very special circumstances,[56] it must remain criminal if it is to be properly controlled, and it must be left to the courts to decide the merits of individual cases.[57]

The effectiveness of the slippery slope argument is in large part due to the nature of the essential legal question regarding assisted suicide, and how that question captures what most concerns many people about the social acceptance of assisted suicide, whether or not it is actually legalized. With respect to the enactment of enabling legislation, the essential question isn't whether there are sometimes good reasons for assisted suicide, much less whether suicide is rational or morally permissible. Instead, the question is what will "flow from" legalization of assisted suicide, and whether those consequences will be bad for society at large regardless of how beneficial they are to some individuals.[58]

Unlike philosophical arguments that suicide is irrational, so assisted suicide is never permissible, and unlike moral prohibitions of both acts, the slippery slope argument appears to make a factual claim about the acceptance or legalization of assisted suicide leading to systematic abuse. This means that evidence should be offered that significant abuse has resulted where assisted suicide has been socially condoned or legalized. Therefore, it also appears that the argument can be countered with empirical evidence, and adherents of assisted suicide are given to citing the Netherlands' fifteen-year experience with sanctioned assisted suicide and contending that it disproves the inevitability of a slide down the slippery slope. But the importance of available empirical evidence for or against the slippery slope argument is actually quite minor. The reasons are that statistics are notoriously pliable and often inconclusive, and the slippery slope argument is not about what may happen because of what has or hasn't already occurred. The argument is really about how we may *change*. As Harvard philosopher Michael Sandel points out, changes in social practices and in law "can bring changes in the way we understand ourselves."[59] In particular, social acceptance and possible legalization of assisted suicide may bring changes that legitimize putting a higher value on "the life that can be lived autonomously and depreciating the life that is dependent."[60] Critics of the slippery slope argument are mistaken to think that it matters overmuch that the number of assisted suicide deaths in the Netherlands hasn't increased markedly. The Dutch experience with condoned assisted suicide is neither temporally extensive nor clear enough to provide a reliable indication of future long-term developments.[61] The real question is whether acceptance—legalized or not—and regular practice of assisted suicide will detrimentally reeducate members of our society to disvalue "life that is dependent." We risk our humanity if we allow the lives of the desperately ill, the very old, or the extremely dependent to be perceived as of little importance and unacceptably burdensome to society. That's why the concern is future-oriented; the question is how acceptance of assisted suicide would "affect policy toward the elderly, the disabled, the poor and the infirm, or reshape the attitudes of doctors toward their ailing patients or children toward their aging parents."[62]

We return to the slippery slope argument in chapter 6. The next chapter gives our criteria for determining when suicide is rational and thus when assisted suicide may be permissible. In chapters 3 through 5 we consider each criterion in turn to clarify the kinds of theoretical and practical factors that need to be balanced against one another in assessing the permissibility of assisted suicide. Of course, dilemmas emerge that we can't hope to resolve. Decisions regarding assisted suicide will remain difficult compromises between the dictates of principle and the entreaties of compassion, and we can only strive for balance between them. The best we can do is to clarify some of those dictates and entreaties as much as possible, given their complexity and diversity, so that some very hard decisions can be made in the most enlightened manner possible.

Summary

Regardless of its legal status, assisted suicide is being practiced now. Ethical guidance is therefore needed prior to resolution of the legal issue, as well as after. But ethical theoreticians too often merely reproduce practical controversies in their diverse theories, while clinicians proceed on a largely *ad hoc* basis in their practices. The deeper reason for the theory-practice gap is that irresolvable conflicts arise between theoretical requirements for permissible assisted suicide and empathic responses to particular cases. Decisions about assisted suicide will always be compromises between these often divergent demands. What is needed is a *balance* of theoretical and practical considerations in making decisions about the permissibility of assisted suicide. The key to achieving that balance is a better understanding that, in the interaction of theory and practice, irresolvable conflicts occur that can be gotten past only through compromise. The two most serious and potentially preclusive obstacles to acceptance of assisted suicide are the claim that suicide is irrational and the slippery slope argument. The first of these is the more fundamental of the two, and in the next chapter, criteria are offered to establish that suicide can be rational.

Notes

1. Most notably Dr. Jack Kevorkian's several trials and Dr. Timothy Quill's case in the United States, and the Sue Rodriguez case in Canada. See the "Media" section of the bibliography.

2. E.g., the reversal in March 1997 of Australia's Northern Territories assisted suicide and voluntary euthanasia legislation. Note that the vote was thirty-eight to thirty-three. See "Australia Strikes Down a State Suicide Law," *New York Times*, March 25, 1997.

3. See Fein 1996; Bruni 1996.

4. Chief Justice William Rehnquist, quoted in Greenhouse 1997b.

5. See Scott 1997.

6. Two basic arguments for decriminalizing assisted suicide appeal: first, the "right to die," as in the constitutional-liberty reasoning of the U.S. Supreme Court's 1992 *Planned Parenthood* v. *Casey* decision, which reiterated women's right to abortion; and second, the equal-protection argument, using the present legality of cessation of life-prolonging treatment. Greenhouse 1996b, 1996c.

7. See Dworkin et al. 1997:41–2; Kolata 1996a, 1997e; Steinfels 1997a; Van Biema 1997.

8. AIDS doctors and oncologists are considerably more prepared to help their patients die than are others. A recent survey showed that 53 percent of AIDS doctors in the San Francisco area had "knowingly prescribed a deadly dose of narcotics to patients who wanted to die" (Van Biema 1997:53).

9. There is, if not a consensus, then something like a common inclination to believe that with respect to legality, "the current system works just fine" in that statutory prohibitions against assisted suicide are generally "loosely enforced" and are "reluctantly violated by doctors when necessary" so that a humane service is provided but kept in check with the threat of severe penalties (Van Biema 1997:53). The trouble is that patients are then entirely dependent on their physicians' particular attitudes toward suicide and assisted suicide. So long as the practice is tacit, patients have no recourse beyond attending clinicians.

10. Kolata 1997e.

11. Here, we follow the common practice of using *ethics* to mean professional conduct-governing principles, as in *medical ethics*, and using *morality* and *moral* to mean cultural and religious principles.

12. Hence the importance to "pro-choice" adherents that a fetus isn't a person and the life in question is the pregnant woman's.

13. Sandel 1997:27.

14. Goodman 1996.

15. Henceforth we refer to physicians, nurses, and other health-care professionals as "clinicians." On the whole, given institutional and professional hierarchies, reference to clinicians' involvement in assisted suicide is usually reference to attending physicians with primary responsibility for treatment decisions. However, this is not always the case, and we don't want to limit ourselves with a too-exclusive term. We collect philosophers, theologians, and other academics as "theoreticians." Hospital-resident clinical ethicists pose a problem, as they are theoreticians with clinical experience and practical duties. As a clinical ethicist, SJT knows full well how difficult it is to keep clinical ethicists

tidily in either the clinical or theoretical category. The distinction between the-oreticians and clinical ethicists has less to do with titles than with day-to-day working contexts. On the whole, we count clinical ethicists with theoreticians, relying on context to suggest when something said about clinicians has some measure of application to clinical ethicists. However, sometimes we need to explicitly include or exclude clinical ethicists in references to clinicians or theoreticians.

16. Dr. Kevorkian is undoubtedly the best known, especially after his 1998 appearance on *60 Minutes*. See "Judge Orders Kevorkian to Be Tried for Murder," *New York Times*, Dec. 10, 1998. Estimates of the number of assisted suicides in which Kevorkian has participated run as high as one hundred. See "Michigan Demands Kevorkian Records," *Kingston Whig-Standard*, July 18, 1998.

17. Most notably, Dr. Henry Morgentaler. See Morgentaler 1982.

18. Kolata 1996a. A key passage is: "[a] survey, by Dr. David A. Asch, an ethicist at the University of Pennsylvania School of Medicine, involved a national sample of 850 nurses who practiced exclusively in adult critical-care units. One hundred forty-one of them said they had received requests from patients or family members to engage in euthanasia or assisted suicide; 129 of the nurses said they had carried out these practices at least once." See also Van Biema 1997. Note that here we refer to cases in which patients request aid in dying; we aren't including those cases in which compassion moves clinicians to delay or avoid treating hopeless cases. For example, CGP was told of a case of a severely hydrocephalic newborn who simply wasn't fed.

19. Attempted suicide and suicide itself are not illegal in most North American and European jurisdictions. Germany decriminalized suicide in 1751, Canada in 1972 (Battin 1992a:46). Figures are sparse, and surveys are compromised by the need to guarantee anonymity, but as noted, estimates are that roughly one in five people requesting assisted suicide get it.

20. Graber and Chassman 1993; Watts and Howell 1992. The basic deter-minants have to do with who is the primary agent and the degrees of awareness and deliberateness involved in the act. The difference may appear overly subtle to some, but it is central to ethical, moral, and legal considerations. We take as a paradigm of *assisted suicide* a case in which a patient requests *the means* to commit suicide: e.g., a prescription for a lethal dose of some sedative or, in more complex cases in which incapacity is a problem, some apparatus that is pro-vided and that the patient can manage to operate. Whatever one may think of Dr. Kevorkian's policies and procedures, his "death machine" *is* operated by the individual requesting assistance in suicide. A paradigm case of voluntary euthanasia is one in which a patient, whether or not physically incapacitated, asks for help in dying but lacks the resolve to commit suicide. In such a case, the patient may ask an attending clinician to administer a fatal dosage of some sedative. In another sort of case, a patient may simply consent to an attending clinician's offer to administer a lethal injection or something of the sort. Things get complicated when what is requested or proposed by a patient or an attending

clinician is cessation of treatment in the form of, say, removal of a ventilator. In some cases, we may want to count requests for cessation of treatment as suicide; in other cases, we may feel it more apt to describe the action taken as voluntary euthanasia. The question is a difficult one, and we have more to say about it, but it is important to distinguish between instances of *self*-killing and instances of consenting to *be* killed. There is, of course, also the possibility of aid in dying being *non*voluntary euthanasia, as when a patient is wholly incapacitated.

21. CGP suspects this happens too often.

22. There are nonterminal situations in which suicide should be permissible because of chronic suffering of either a physical or a psychological sort. For consideration of *preemptive* suicide, see Prado 1990.

23. We strongly disagree with the view that "[i]n an ideal world," the courts would leave the issue of assisted suicide alone to allow "the space and time for the moral reflection that the issue demands" (Carter 1996:29). Assisted suicide is a present reality.

24. CGP had one graduate student who was consumed by the issue of the permissibility of abortion but insisted on reading only contributors to the debate whom she knew to be Catholic, on the grounds that she "didn't trust" other contributors. Her response to questions about understanding opposing views was that the contributors she read reviewed counterarguments in making their own. Clearly, the question of trust extended to the assumption that opposing views would be impartially presented.

25. See Kolata 1997b. The trouble with such reliance is that either accounts of case studies remain anecdotal, and so of dubious value in application to new cases, or clinicians are themselves theorizing in trying to derive general principles from case studies. The only thing that would seem to justify such inefficient duplication of labor is the dubious conviction that only someone with ongoing firsthand experience can successfully draw general principles from case studies.

26. Including clinical ethicists.

27. This approach is more than evident in the literature aimed at clinicians. See, for example, the much-read *Ethics in Nursing* (Benjamin and Curtis 1986).

28. As will emerge, many clinicians ignore or dismiss the often elusive but still important difference between requested cessation of treatment and suicide.

29. For some, theoretical work *begins* with the assumption that suicide is irrational and always wrong, hence assisted suicide is never permissible. See Donnelly 1978:89–95.

30. It is too large a question to pursue here, but basically, scientific theory *enables* technological advances, as theorizing about lift led to the design of airplane wings. Ethical theory is more a matter of *discernment* of applicable principles operant in what we more or less intuitively accept as proper action.

31. Because of the gender issue, and to avoid the repetitiveness of "his or her" and "she or he," we adopt the increasingly common use of the plurals "their" and "they" in singular constructions.

32. Including clinical ethicists.

33. Admittedly, not all clinicians feel it necessary to do anything outside the boundaries set by general principles. We owe this reminder to Margaret Battin.

34. The connection is apparently not obvious to all. The point is that only if suicide is judged rational is it permissible to facilitate it. The alternatives are either to perform some form of euthanasia (i.e., nonvoluntary when the person in question is in irremediable agony but not capable of making an autonomous decision) or to be immorally and perhaps criminally complicitous in the commission of an irrational self-destructive act.

35. Recall that we're using *ethical* to refer to professional principles of conduct and *moral* to refer to broader principles of conduct.

36 . See Toulmin 1989.

37. This is a question that Aristotle addressed in reminding us that in practical reasoning we can't demand greater precision than the subject matter allows. Toulmin 1989:48–9.

38. See Battin 1990:5–6.

39. Berger 1987, quoted in Code 1994:83. We define the technical sense more carefully later.

40. Gilligan 1982:19.

41. We have in mind physical incapacity, such as paralysis. Psychological incapacity could possibly merit assistance in suicide, but such incapacity seems to cast doubt on the agent's intentions.

42. Rationality is no longer unproblematic. Philosophers such as Richard Rorty and Michel Foucault claim that rationality is wholly historical and parochial instead of timeless and universal. But by "rational" we mean only what is in conformity with accepted standards of reasoning. In this sense, "rational" is whatever contrasts with assessment of decisions or actions as pathological or unwitting. We return to this matter in the next chapter.

43. The idea here is that obligations are valued or devalued in being acknowledged or rejected. Assessment of whether obligations preclude suicide comes down to deciding whether meeting obligations is valued enough to prevent suicide.

44. Claims that suicide is aberrant run from suicide being against God's law, to suicide being a result of psychopathological or unbearable emotional influences, to suicidal decisions being irrational because we can't understand what it is to be dead and so can't rationally choose to die. Prado 1990:114–6.

45. Roy, Williams, and Dickens 1994:412.

46. It is mainly non-Christian moral codes that allow suicide, as in the case of *seppuku* or *hara-kiri*, but we are past the time when it could be argued that Christian morality is the only true morality. See Prado 1990:79–96. And despite Christian culture's negative view of suicide, our own pre-Christian history contains numerous examples of honorable suicide, such as Socrates, Cato, Seneca, Brutus, and, more marginally within that culture, Boadicea, Hannibal, and the hundreds at Masada.

47. Moral and religious codes may concede that it can be in an individual's own interests to commit suicide but still prohibit it as violating some principle or harming the greatest number or because life is God's gift.

48. Ayer and O'Grady 1992:197.

49. Perhaps we should add "in a given culture."

50. Compare a clinician's situation regarding abortion. There could be a medical and/or professional duty to abort a fetus, but a moral prohibition to doing so.

51. There are thorny issues about responsibilities and duties to patients. Clinicians' personal moral and religious beliefs need to be taken into account in cases of assisting suicide, as is now usually done with abortion. Against this, basic humanity may require aid in dying when suffering is intense enough, regardless of the beliefs of attending clinicians.

52. Sanctioning assisted suicide needn't involve legalization. Those assisting suicide may not be charged; or if charged, not prosecuted; or if charged and prosecuted, not convicted.

53. Interview with Dr. Arthur Caplan on "The Kevorkian Verdict," *Frontline*, broadcast May 14, 1996. See also Kaveny and Langan 1996.

54. See, e.g., Burgess 1993; Devettere 1992; Dresser and Whitehouse 1994; Freedman 1992 (reply to van der Burg 1992); Howe 1992; Ogilvie and Potts 1994; Tallis 1996; van der Burg 1992.

55. Wilkes 1996:22.

56. What some deem special enough circumstances to justify assisted suicide are, in effect, circumstances that warrant not assisted suicide but voluntary or nonvoluntary euthanasia.

57. The argument is lent force when assisted suicide and euthanasia are confused by neglect of the crucial difference between helping someone to die who chooses to but cannot do so alone and killing someone.

58. Some believe that U.S. courts have already jeopardized the social good by "invent[ing], out of thin air, a right to die" (Rosen 1996:cover).

59. Sandel 1997, quoted in Steinfels 1997a:12.

60. Steinfels 1997a:12. As Sandel (1997:27) puts it:

Existing laws against assisted suicide reflect and entrench certain views about what gives life meaning. But the same would be true were the Court to declare, in the name of autonomy, a right to assisted suicide. The new regime would not simply expand the range of options, but would encourage the tendency to view life less as a gift and more as a possession. It might heighten the prestige we accord autonomous, independent lives and depreciate the claims of those seen to be dependent.

61. For one thing, the Netherlands has a notably homogeneous and relatively small population, where tacit understandings can be relied on to work considerably better than in larger, more culturally diverse populations.

62. Sandel 1997:27.

2

CRITERIA FOR RATIONAL SUICIDE

The *Dictionary of Modern Thought* assures us that someone's suicide "may be regarded as rational" if that individual "prefers death to any other possible future."[1] And the *New York Times* assured millions of readers that "the concept of rational suicide is gaining credence."[2] Nonetheless, our culture's prevalent view, which has obvious biological roots, is that life is the ultimate value, and most people take it "as an article of commonsensism" that self-destruction isn't rational.[3] A more sophisticated view is that because life is the precondition of all value, it is irrational to abandon it until value becomes irrevocably unattainable.[4] But it is rarely acknowledged that value has become irrevocably unattainable. Even in the direst circumstances, people continue to believe that things are never so hopeless as to make committing suicide the sensible thing to do. For the most part, then, suicide is seldom conceded to be rational and is usually viewed as "the product of mental illness," or its attempt as "a desperate dangerous 'cry for help' used by someone who does not really want to die."[5]

However, Margaret Battin is quite right in holding that in "the absence of any compelling evidence to the contrary," we have to accept that someone may choose to abandon life "on the basis of reasoning which is by all usual standards adequate."[6] There are times when it is rational[7] to prefer dying to living in a manner considered intolerable. Our culture must come more widely to acknowledge that sometimes suicide does make sense and to respect someone's choice to abandon life.[8] With that acknowledgment and respect must come acceptance that helping

31

someone who is incapacitated to commit suicide shouldn't always be a
criminal act.

The way to enable the needed acknowledgment that suicide can be
rational is to state clearly under what conditions it makes good sense to
end one's own life. As said in chapter 1, that is when choosing to commit
suicide is in keeping with sound reasoning, is in the best interests of the
person involved, and is in line with that person's values.[9] The main purpose of this chapter is to formulate these conditions as criteria for
rational suicide and to explain enough about them to proceed with a
more detailed consideration of each. But as is always the case in philosophy, terms need to be defined; we first need to specify precisely what
the criteria apply *to*. At this point, we also need to ask the reader's indul-
gence, as the balance of this chapter requires careful treatment of a
number of abstract points.

DEFINING SUICIDE AND ASSISTED SUICIDE

The *Oxford Companion to Philosophy* tells us that "the most conventional definition of 'suicide' is intentionally caused self destruction."[10]
The trouble with defining *suicide*[11] as self-destruction or self-*killing* is
that many define suicide as self-*murder*. That is, many hold that the act
of taking one's own life is never justified and so is intrinsically morally
wrong.[12] But suicide can't be made morally wrong by definition. So long
as there is no universal moral ban on suicide, defining suicide as self-
murder illegitimately stipulates its moral status while ignoring exceptions.[13] Suicide may be prohibited by particular moral codes and defined
as immoral within those codes, but barring universal prohibition it must
be recognized that some moral codes allow suicide as justified self-
killing. Our preliminary definitions of suicide and assisted suicide, then,
are as morally neutral *self-killing* and *self-killing with help*. These are
the acts to be assessed as rational or irrational. Assessment of those acts
as moral or immoral is a separate, subordinate question, because an act
can be moral or immoral only if it's rational, since only a rational act can
be a *responsible* act. Moral assessment of an act also requires specification of the operant moral code.

More pertinent difficulties with defining suicide are posed by "sacri-
ficial death, martyrdom that could have been avoided, actions that risk

near-certain death, . . . addiction-induced overdosing, coercion to self-caused death," and, of particular concern to us, "refusals of medical treatment with foreknowledge of death."[14] For our purposes, the definition of suicide has to allow for or exclude these problematic cases in which individual autonomy is in some way qualified. Defining suicide for our purposes requires that we begin with the class of all self-killings, including those in which death occurs partly as a consequence of the agents' deliberate actions but also partly as a result of factors not under their control.[15] We then narrow the focus to include only those cases within the larger class that are full-fledged self-killings, in the sense that agents are solely responsible for their own deaths and the self-destructive acts are done, in legal terms, "with intent" to die.[16] To define this sort of self-destruction we adopt Tom L. Beauchamp's definition of suicide, which holds that "[a] person commits suicide if: (1) that person intentionally brings about his or her own death; (2) others do not coerce him or her to do the action;[17] and (3) death is caused by conditions arranged by the person for the purpose of bringing about his or her own death."[18]

Fortunately, Beauchamp's definition doesn't need revision to cover assisted suicide. His third requirement amply covers the actions of others who uncoercively assist suicide.[19] The key clause is "conditions arranged by the person." The conditions arranged can include the actions of others. The only proviso is that those actions are at the agent's explicit behest and instruction. But while Beauchamp's definition covers assisted suicide, it needs amplification for the sake of clarity. Two points need to be made explicit: one about the requirement that suicide be intentional, the other about how Beauchamp's third requirement covers assisted suicide.

Beauchamp's requirement that suicide be intentional must be understood to mean that the act is done with adequate comprehension or "vivid awareness" of consequences.[20] Without vivid awareness of the consequences,[21] an act can't be fully intentional, so there can be no question of permissible assistance in its commission if that awareness is lacking. Only if suicide is intentional in this fully aware sense can it be entirely responsible, and only if it is a responsible act can another person rightfully participate in its commission. In what follows, *intentional* will be understood as carrying this sense of awareness of consequences.

The second amplification has to do with preserving the distinction between assisted suicide and euthanasia. In cases in which an individual is being treated by clinicians, assisted *suicide* requires that the individual not die as a result of unsolicited actions by those clinicians. The request for assistance in suicide must be explicit, and, when possible, the patient in question must play an active, primary role. As we will see, mere expression of a wish not to go on living or for cessation of life-supporting treatment isn't enough for assisted suicide. If clinicians act on such an expression, they may be performing compassionate voluntary euthanasia,[22] but they wouldn't be assisting suicide.[23] Given that a person who is hospitalized or otherwise under medical care is regularly medicated by others and is usually almost entirely dependent on them, it is necessary to spell out that to be assisted suicide, death must be caused by conditions deliberately and knowingly "arranged by the person for the purpose of bringing about his or her own death."

Suicide, then, is understood as intentional, uncoerced (morally neutral) self-killing by one's own action. Assisted suicide is understood as the commission of suicide, as defined, with the equally intentional and uncoerced help of another. With suicide defined, we must focus more narrowly on those cases in which intentional and uncoerced self-killing is done with intent and by a person competent[24] to decide to commit suicide.[25] Our criteria for rational suicide apply to this narrowest subclass of self-destructive acts.

CRITERIA FOR RATIONAL SUICIDE

The criteria offered here are criteria for telling when suicide is rational; they determine when suicide is the most rational means, in the sense of the most effective instrumentality, to achieve what best serves a person's values and interests.[26] Jacques Choron provides a good place to start articulating the criteria, arguing that suicide is rational if the suicidist's motives "seem justifiable, or at least 'understandable,' by the majority of his contemporaries in the same culture or social group."[27] Choron, like Battin, locates the rationality of suicide not in the context of philosophical absolutes but in the context of established standards.[28] His point is that suicidal reasoning must have similar force for cultural and social peers as for the suicidist, though they may reject its conclusion, e.g., because of moral prohibitions.

Choron's acceptance of understanding as sufficient, when justification is not attainable, challenges the adequacy of the theoretically favored perspective of the detached observer. This is because reference to motives being understandable to peers, even if not wholly justifiable,

goes beyond the assessment of suicidal motives by abstract requirements. It clearly calls for some effort at empathic understanding of an
individual's suicidal motives in terms of that individual's singular situation. Choron's point is that only if there is reasonable effort at such
understanding can it be judged that a potential suicidist's motives aren't
rational and may be pathological or otherwise suspect. Otherwise, those
judgments would be made entirely on the basis of abstract requirements
which might or might not be adequate to the particular circumstances.[29]
The key element Choron provides, then, is the necessity of peers finding
suicidal motivation cogent, something that requires empathic understanding of the suicidist's particular situation.

Battin also provides key elements for our criteria. She gives her own
criteria for rational suicide in two groups. The first, her "nonimpairment" group, includes the "ability to reason, [a] realistic world view, and
adequacy of information." These three conditions have to do with the
proper conduct of suicidal deliberation. The second, or "satisfaction of
interests" group includes, "avoidance of harm and accordance with fundamental interests." These two conditions have to do with what suicide
is supposed to achieve. Battin sums up by saying that "[w]e typically
speak of a decision as 'rational' . . . if it is made in an unimpaired way;
we also speak of a decision as 'rational' . . . if it satisfies [the agent's]
interests."[30]

While the requirement for a realistic worldview needs further discussion, it is uncontroversial that suicidal deliberation must be free of impairment due to muddled reasoning, false information, or ignorance, though,
as we will see, this may be a matter of degree. We could not allow a person
to commit suicide while demented or confused,[31] while wrongly believing
that they had a terminal illness, or while unaware of important facts
directly pertinent to their situation. What is more problematic is the matter
of avoidance of harm and accordance with interests. The force of most
arguments against the rationality of suicide is precisely that suicide is
always the worst possible self-inflicted harm and so can never be in one's
interests.[32] Against this, Battin argues that in assessing whether one harms
oneself in committing suicide to avoid something unbearable, we have to
look at "the amount of other experience permitted . . . and whether this
other experience is of intrinsic value."[33] Assessment of whether suicide is
in or against one's interests is a matter of assessing what must be borne in
continuing to live, and whether its being borne is made worthwhile by
"important experience during the pain-free intervals."[34]

Battin is largely right, but there's a problem about accordance of suicide with fundamental interests. To clarify, we need to draw a somewhat

artificial distinction between interests and values. This is a distinction we've anticipated in speaking of both values and interests. Value, i.e., worth or merit, is what determines interests. What is of value is in one's interests, and the greater the value, the greater the interest. This much seems clear. But it is commonly thought that life's supposedly incomparable value generates so great an interest in survival that it overrides any contrary values. The result is a pronounced tendency on the part of clinicians, and the public at large, to heavily discount an individual's values when those values prompt a decision to abandon life.[35] Someone's conclusion that dying is in their interests, because it accords with their values, is usually seen as confused or more likely as being caused by transient desperation. When the interest in survival and other values conflict, many believe that the conflict must be due to misguided favoring of those other values, because they find it incomprehensible that it could be in someone's interests to die and so lose what is supposedly of greatest value.

But if value determines interests, what must be remembered is that it is what *we* value that determines our interests. It is a mistake to think that survival generates an objective value that is independent of what particular individuals prize. If we are to understand how suicide may be rational, we have to keep in mind the personal or subjective[36] character of values and interests. That subjectivity is evident in the interplay of values and interests in suicidal deliberation, which is more complex than simple opposition of the interest in survival to other values. The cases that get attention are those in which people choose not to live because they value something else more than their own survival. But individuals may endure torment, which it is very much in their interests to escape, and *not* commit suicide because of the value they put on a moral code or religious faith that prohibits suicide. In other words, suicide may be avoided not because it is always in one's interests to survive but because other values outweigh *its* value. People can value survival for reasons other than that it is survival. This shows that survival can be the object of evaluative assessment and deliberation, and therefore that it can sometimes be subordinated to other values, as well as sometimes override them. In fact, the ability to value something more than personal survival partly defines what it is to be rational. This is a point argued by philosopher Richard Rorty.

Rorty defines rationality as three distinct but overlapping abilities. It is the second of these that is relevant here, and that is the ability to "establish an evaluative hierarchy" and so the capacity to "set goals other than mere survival."[37] Rationality, then, has to do in part with establishing priorities, and that may include not only giving priority to something over one's own survival but also setting conditions on what is acceptable survival.[38] Suicide prompted by terminal illness or other health crises can be rational because it is possible for people to value quality of life more than continuing to live. And regardless of how odd it may sound, when people do put a higher value on something other than their own survival, it is in their interests to die. One obvious sort of case is when the value that members of a particular culture put on honor or atonement makes it more in their interests to commit suicide than to live in shame.[39]

The requirement that, to be rational, suicide must accord with "fundamental interests," then, is not sufficiently fine-grained. Unqualified reference to fundamental interests is too broad, because even what is ordinarily our most basic interest in survival may conflict with deeply held values that generate competing and perhaps overriding interests. Our criteria need to balance the requirement that suicide accord with the interests we normally share as human beings, with a requirement that suicide be in accordance with the values that define us as individuals.

We have, then, four preliminary conditions for rational suicide: that suicide be intentional and uncoerced (Beauchamp), that motivation be understandable and cogent (Choron), that there be no impairment in reasoning (Battin), and that suicide be consistent with interests (Battin). These conditions are insufficient to establish the rationality of suicide as they stand; they need to be reformulated and complemented with reference to the accordance of suicide with values. There is also a need to ensure that suicide is a genuine option for the individual, in the sense that it is felt to be a compelling possibility and is considered willfully and determinedly. There is a marked danger that suicide might be impetuously or unreflectively committed under what Elizabeth Kristol calls a "soothing moral shroud."[40] This happens when desperate but irresolute individuals convince themselves that "an expert we ... entrust with a wide range of decisions regarding our well-being"[41] believes that they should commit suicide. An attending clinician may inadvertently[42] provide "an escape from the burden of autonomous choice" by unintentionally offering terminal patients "a tantalizing opportunity to escape ... paralyzing doubt." For instance, a clinician may review a patient's various options and mention assisted suicide in the process.[43] Some patients may hastily fasten on the clinician's remarks as a way out of their predicament. The attraction of seeing suicide as *proposed to them* rather than something they choose themselves is that "the ultimate responsibility for taking one's life [is] shared. More than shared, it [is] validated by a doctor."[44] Our criteria must exclude cases in which this sort of thing occurs, making suicide significantly less than an autonomous choice.[45]

Mention of autonomy requires articulation of one of its implicit aspects that is central to our criteria for rational suicide. The criteria have to do with suicide being rational when it is the best means to resolve a medical crisis. As noted earlier, the criteria apply only to suicide that is intentional and uncoerced, which means suicide that is done autonomously in the sense of freely, resolutely, and with full knowledge of what one is doing. However, one can act autonomously and do so without due reflection. On those occasions we act resolutely and freely and with full or at least adequate knowledge of what we're doing at the time, but without thinking through the implications of what we do or why we do what we do.[46] If suicide is an autonomous act only in this ordinary sense, it may not be rational, because the gravity of the act requires more.

Webster's Unabridged Dictionary provides the missing element that, though implicit in the concept of autonomy, is often overlooked because *autonomous* usually means only "independent" or "free." The implicit element is vital to the rationality of suicide and is given as "(3) the right of the individual to govern himself *according to . . . reason.*"[47] Autonomous action is not only free; it is action whose implications and consequences are for the best, given the agent's values and interests.[48] To be fully autonomous, then, an act must be thought out and its consequences and implications understood and accepted. Autonomous acts contrast not only with unintentional or coerced behavior but also with behavior that, while free, is to some degree unthinking or impulsive. Acts done unthinkingly or impulsively, even if autonomous, may not be in keeping with reason if unintended and undesired consequences are detrimental to the agent's interests and values. From here on, when we speak of suicide as autonomous, we mean an act done knowingly, resolutely, freely, and according to good reason.[49]

We can now give our criteria. The criteria specify conditions having to do with reasoning, motivation, and interests. They don't include specification of autonomy, because they apply only to autonomous self-killing. The requirement that suicide be autonomous self-killing is a precondition and not itself a criterion. Part of the significance of this point has to do with maintaining the distinction between assisted suicide and various forms of euthanasia. When we are dealing with cases in which individuals for some reason aren't capable of autonomous action,[50] the issue is whether or not to perform nonvoluntary[51] euthanasia, not whether or not to assist in the commission of suicide. Our criteria apply to those cases only in an extended way, mainly in that they apply to surrogates' deliberations and decisions. More complex are cases of individuals who request voluntary euthanasia but are unwilling to take part in causing their own deaths. In these cases, the criteria apply to those individuals' deliberations and decisions, *as well as* to the deliberations and decisions of clinicians performing euthanasia. This is because those clinicians are the primary agents in causing death in the provision of voluntary euthanasia.

Suicide, then, assuming that it is autonomous self-killing, is a rational act when

1. suicide is a genuine option for the agent, chosen after deliberation consistent with accepted standards of reasoning and unimpaired by error, false beliefs, or lack of relevant information; *and*

2. the agent's motivating values are cogent to others, not unduly contravening the agent's interests; *and*

3. suicide is in the agent's interests, not causing more harm than continuing to live.[52]

THE USUAL COMPLICATIONS

We have to clarify a number of points before considering the criteria individually. The first is that we acknowledge that the criteria will look too demanding to many. Many clinical ethicists and most clinicians will think that the criteria articulate an ideal that can only be approached. Contrary to this, most theoreticians will think that self-destruction must meet stringent conditions to be rational, and especially to merit someone else's involvement. Their view is that the entanglements of practical experience shouldn't be allowed to soften those conditions. Both views pose problems. The main difficulty with the view that the criteria describe an ideal and must be contextually interpreted is how to effectively regulate and standardize their application while allowing for significant interpretive latitude. The main difficulty with the view that the criteria need strict application is that "[p]erhaps none of our acts are ever *wholly* rational," since human actions "are never wholly free from emotion, training, circumstantial coercion, or other arational components."[53] Our clarification is that provision of the criteria doesn't of itself prejudge whether or to what degree they may be qualified in their application.

A second clarification is that, at most, the criteria give the necessary conditions for rational suicide, but not sufficient conditions. Even if completely satisfied, the criteria don't make suicide compulsory. There is always a difference between what sound reasoning says individuals *should* do and what they *choose* to do. Recall Hume's insight that "[r]eason is, and ought only to be the slave of the passions, and can never pretend to any other office than to serve and obey them."[54] What we offer are criteria to determine when suicide is rational, hence permissible and well-advised. If suicide is the wisest choice in some circumstances, we may fail to understand someone's unwillingness to take that course of action, but if they choose to live regardless of the suffering that entails, it is their choice.

Third, some cases of what is described as assisted suicide in medical contexts are problematic. Patients who ask for help in committing suicide may raise questions about their rationality, but not about their intentions. In contrast, patients who request cessation of life-sustaining treatment do raise questions about their intentions. It is a difficult thing to establish that patients both fully understand and intend the fatal consequences of cessation of treatment.[55] Because our criteria apply to autonomous self-killing, in order for patients to commit suicide by requesting cessation of treatment, they must understand and intend that death will result from accession to the request.[56]

A fourth clarification has to do with how most clinicians don't accept that their own present practices regarding some cases of requested cessation of treatment are properly described as assisting at suicide.[57] Death resulting from such requests is thought to be the inevitable effect of an underlying condition. Cessation of life-sustaining treatment is perceived as merely letting nature take its course, not as an act contributing to the death of the patient. Many clinicians may feel that our criteria don't apply to requested cessation of treatment. But many theoreticians and clinical ethicists see this as an evasion or rationalization prompted by moral misgivings.[58] Requested cessation of treatment clearly seems to be assisted suicide in a significant number of instances. If patients are entirely incapacitated,[59] the only self-destructive act they may be capable of is to request cessation of treatment.[60] Not describing some cases of requested cessation of life-sustaining treatment as assisted suicide seems to be a semantic issue, not a conceptual, legal, or moral one.

There are two reasons why description of present practices is important: First, our criteria apply to present practices, not to proposed new practices of assisted suicide. Consideration of the criteria, then, is a matter of deliberating what clinicians currently do, not what they might do if assisted suicide becomes a sanctioned option. In order that effective ethical guidance be possible, clinicians must acknowledge that many of them are assisting suicide *now,* and not only considering how they'll conduct themselves if asked to do so at some future time. Second, requested cessation of treatment is presently legal,[61] even if the results are known to be fatal, and is regularly done in our hospitals. If requested cessation of treatment is assisted suicide in some cases, then those cases of requested cessation of treatment are presently cases of *de facto* legal assisted suicide.

A fifth clarification has to do with the differences between assisted suicide and voluntary euthanasia. By *euthanasia,* the ancient Greeks meant simply "a good or easy death."[62] During the last century, the word came to mean death caused by someone else in the best interests of a suffering individual. Until fairly recently, euthanasia was characterized in the bioethics literature as either "active" euthanasia, defined as deliberate killing of someone for merciful reasons, or "passive" euthanasia, defined as someone being "allowed to die" by either cessation or noninitiation of treatment. Euthanasia was also described as "voluntary," "involuntary," or "nonvoluntary,"[63] depending on the degree of consent and of awareness on the part of the patient. Currently the consensus among clinicians is that withholding or withdrawing life-sustaining treatment does "not involve euthanasia at all but merely good medical practice," because at some point "treatment is not beneficial" and continuing it "merely prolongs dying."[64] *Euthanasia* now refers more narrowly to "the act of ending the life of a person, from compassionate motives, when he is already terminally ill or when his suffering has become unbearable."[65] The important implication for us is that if cessation of treatment isn't passive euthanasia but a judgment call about treatment effectiveness, then it seems that clinicians' involvement in a patient's willing but nonnatural death must be either assisted suicide or voluntary euthanasia.

In the courts, the difference between assisted suicide, in which the patient is the primary agent, and voluntary euthanasia, in which a clinician is the primary agent, is thought to be clear, in principle, and is usually crucial in particular cases. But with respect to application of our criteria, things are more complicated. The trouble is that some cases of euthanasia are "a sort of other-assisted suicide."[66] The distinction between assisted suicide and voluntary euthanasia is one of degree and perspective. The fact is that there are *two* agents involved in assisted suicide. Given this duality, the difference between assisted suicide and euthanasia is a subtle one of who is or becomes the primary or dominant agent.[67] It must be borne in mind that our criteria apply to the deliberation and action of the suicidist as the primary agent. Any erosion of that primacy violates the precondition that suicide be an autonomous act. At the same time, the criteria also apply to whoever assists suicide. It isn't sufficient that suicide be rational from the agent's point of view to make assisting it permissible. The person assisting has to follow the reasoning and find it cogent, because in assisting suicide they are, in the sense just mentioned, performing voluntary euthanasia. Ideally, a person assisting suicide is only an instrument of another's will. But we can't simply be instruments, since we have individual rational, ethical, moral, and practical obligations regarding our conduct. Someone assisting suicide, then, may do so only when the criteria are satisfied both from the suicidist's point of view and from their own. And since no one can act purely as an instrument, in assisting the commission of suicide, one performs voluntary euthanasia to the extent that it's one's own actions that cause death.

A last clarification has to do with rationality or what governs sound reasoning. As pointed out earlier, Choron and Battin locate the question of the rationality of suicide in the domain of established cultural standards, rather than attempting to give a philosophically definitive account of the nature of rationality. This is important, because postmodern philosophers have made the notion of rationality a problematic one by criticizing the traditional conception of rationality as "ahistorical" and independent of social practices. Rejecting a tradition as old as Plato that human beings embody an objective rationality, Rorty and French philosopher Michel Foucault spearheaded the reconception of rationality as a product of historical practices and values.[68] We obviously can't hope to resolve a major current philosophical debate in advancing our project, but we don't need to. By rationality, we mean historically established standards of reasoning. Our main concern with rationality is not with its nature but with rebutting the claim that suicide is irrational by current standards.[69] Therefore we follow Choron and Battin and rely on "reasoning which is *by all usual standards* adequate."[70] Whether those standards are universal or not, timeless or not, aren't questions we need to take up.

SUMMARY

The claim that suicide is irrational can be rebutted by establishing that suicide is rational when it is an autonomous act, when its deliberation conforms to established reasoning standards, and when it best serves the suicidist's values and interests. Three criteria applying only to autonomous self-killing are provided, covering (1) the genuineness and nonimpaired nature of a suicidal decision, (2) the cogency of motivation and suicide's accordance with the person's value-priorities in relation to fundamental interests, and (3) suicide's accordance with the person's interests. Moral prohibitions are not preclusive of suicide, since rational suicide does not violate a universal prohibition. If suicide may be rational and is not precluded by moral prohibition, assisted suicide may be permissible. Our use of *rational* and *rationality* appeals to established standards, not to a particular philosophical conception of rationality. The major question that the criteria raise for us is the extent to which they require strict application or admit of contextual interpretation and qualification.

NOTES

1. Bullock, Stallybrass, and Trombley 1988:721. "Prefers death" is a misleading expression, because what is preferred is not death but rather not continuing to live in the relevant circumstances.
2. Tolchin 1989.
3. Donnelly 1978:89.
4. See Hook 1988.
5. Battin 1984:297.
6. Battin 1984:301.
7. To repeat, suicide is rational when it is the best means to achieve the best purpose, where "best means" is the action that sound reasoning determines to be optimal, and "best purpose" is what is most beneficial to an individual's interests and values.
8. A loved one's emotional pressure can be as imprisoning as any doctor's overly diligent efforts to prolong life.
9. We clarify later why interests and values need to be distinguished.
10. Honderich 1995:859.

11. Caramuel coined the word *suicidium* in his *Theologia Moralis Fundamentalis* in the seventeenth century (Van Hoof 1960:163).

12. Those categorically against suicide hold that it is always unjustified killing, thus murder (Donnelly 1978:89–95). When Sir William Blackstone codified English law in the eighteenth century, he held suicide to be self-murder and a felony (Honderich 1995:859).

13. Note that even if it is argued that there is only one universal moral code for all human beings, and that diversity of moral codes is due to error and lack of discernment, it would still be open to question whether that universal code prohibits suicide.

14. Honderich 1995:859.

15. High-risk acts, refusals of treatment with hope of survival, and martyrdom are included in this group.

16. Assistance in suicide doesn't violate this condition; what is ruled out is another's act or an event not under the agent's control contributing to the agent's death. Intent excludes hope of survival. However, faith in an afterlife is a complicating factor.

17. Coercion doesn't mean only force; it includes such things as reminders of the cost of maintaining life and the cumulative effect their repetition may have. But there is a sense in which the sort of suicide that concerns us is not wholly uncoerced, because it is committed to end or avoid an intolerable situation.

18. Beauchamp 1980:77, quoted in Rachels 1986:81.

19. The criterion has other applications, such as when someone attempts suicide but dies as a result of an extraneous cause.

20. Harman 1986:2.

21. Belief in an afterlife complicates this condition, but what needs to be ruled out is not so much specific beliefs regarding survival as much as a lack of understanding of at least possible annihilatory consequences. Freud may be right that "the human unconsciousness 'believes itself immortal'" (Battin 1984:299). But it is likelier that someone may commit suicide while avoiding full realization of the consequences.

22. They may even be performing non- or involuntary euthanasia if, say, the patient's expressed desire wasn't well thought out or was only the expression of a wish that their suffering would end.

23. Again, the important difference is *who is the primary agent.*

24. This isn't the "expertise" sense of *competence*; it is the "capability" sense used when we say that individuals are "not competent" and mean that they are unable to make major decisions or care for themselves. Under current law, one considering suicide is presumed incompetent in this sense and can be detained in a psychiatric facility. Also, a psychiatric consultation is one of the first things done on admission to hospital after a suicide attempt. Lifton 1987:221.

25. Here we rule out cases in which someone intentionally commits suicide, and whose death results from their own actions, but who is driven to suicide by despondency, compulsion, and so forth.

26. Compare Quill, Cassel, and Meier 1992.

27. Choron 1972:96–7.

28. Battin 1982:301.

29. Even Aquinas didn't think that was good enough in the case of judging sin. In defining natural law and "case morality," he required that confessors take into account *peccatoris circumstantiae atque peccati*: "the circumstances both of the sinner and of the sin" (Toulmin 1989:48).

30. Battin 1982:289. Battin is also concerned with whether a person understands the consequences of suicide, but she sees the issue as a purely psychological one. See Battin 1984:299.

31. Regardless of how firm the underlying beliefs, there are some things we won't accept as reasons for suicide. A good example of a "confused" reason for suicide was the Heaven's Gate group's belief that the appearance of the Hale-Bopp comet in March 1997 was a sign that members of the group had to kill themselves to be rid of their physical bodies in order to be taken to heaven in the comet. See Purdum 1997; Niebuhr 1997; Bruni 1997.

32. The law allows interference with attempted suicide, described as prevention of self-inflicted harm, as a defense against charges incurred in the process of interfering. "[S]ociety has nearly as strong an . . . interest in thwarting suicide as it does in thwarting murder" (Robinson 1984:193). Individuals' personal autonomy to commit suicide is "dismissed" in law (Robinson 1984:193; compare Shipp 1988).

33. Battin 1984:312.

34. Battin 1984:312.

35. Some clinicians are often at a loss to understand how people can allow certain values to jeopardize their interest in survival, e.g., by forbidding a necessary blood transfusion.

36. Unfortunately, "subjective" now connotes relativism. We don't intend it in that sense and mean only that a person's values and interests are ultimately determined by the individual and not by nature or society.

37. The other abilities are "the ability to cope with the environment" and the "ability not to be overly disconcerted by difference from oneself, not to respond aggressively to such differences (Rorty 1992:581).

38. In the first case, individuals may sacrifice their lives for loved ones; in the second case, they may be unwilling to endure life as, e.g., paraplegics.

39. See Prado 1990:79–97.

40. Kristol 1993.

41. Kristol 1993.

42. Of course, some may quite intentionally encourage a patient to commit suicide in very special circumstances.

43. This is a hard call. Even if assisted suicide were legal and an available treatment option, we are uncertain whether attending clinicians should mention it as an option. To many patients, the mere mention of assisted suicide as a possible course of action could appear to be a suggestion or a proposed solution

carrying all the weight of medical expertise. Later, we consider the vulnerability of patients to be influenced by clinicians, but there's no question that clinicians can't simply review patients' options without running the risk of being taken to be *endorsing* one or another. This is especially true of a measure as desperate as suicide. Mere mention of suicide as an option could be wrongly heard by a patient as a dire warning of fearsome and untreatable suffering to come that would be best avoided by self-destruction.

44. Kristol 1993.

45. We're very much aware that the capacity for autonomous decisions is jeopardized and qualified by patient suffering. There's no question that a healthy individual's ability to act autonomously differs significantly from that of someone enduring great stress and pain. One of us knows a physician who takes this as simply precluding the need to get any sort of concurrence from some patients regarding their treatment. However, as in the case of rationality, we aren't appealing to a metaphysical absolute. In speaking of autonomy in the relevant cases, we appeal to what reflective consensus would judge to be acts or decisions best described as the patients' own, as opposed to ones imposed on them or assumed on their behalf or even ones that they may be manipulated into making.

46. Note that in law we are held responsible for acts judged to be autonomous, even if they are done without due reflection. It's also worth noting that when we do something without proper reflection and are challenged as to why we did what we did, we usually claim autonomy to divert or preclude the need to give reasons.

47. Second edition (1983:128), our emphasis.

48. Some may wonder why a tight connection is assumed between something being rational or according to reason and it being for the best or the right thing. The basic sense of *rational* is instrumental: That is rational which most effectively achieves a desired objective, whatever that may be. Although what is or isn't the best objective may be arguable, it isn't arguable that reason is all about how to get what we want. This is Hume's point in saying that reason can only serve the passions. Without desired objectives, action is neither rational nor otherwise in the instrumental sense.

49. Recall that we include vivid awareness of consequences in speaking of intentional action and in speaking of autonomous action. Note also that the deontological principle of autonomy, respect for persons' free choices, needs no emendation, because it presupposes that the free choices that are to be respected are autonomous in the relevant sense. The principle, being Kantian, applies only to reasoned choices.

50. For instance, patients may be too distracted by constant severe pain or may be comatose.

51. Here we're thinking of cases of comatose patients. It's conceivable that there might be cases of rational and permissible *involuntary* euthanasia. For instance, some suffering individuals may be competent enough to reject euthanasia but not competent enough to understand why it would be in their

best interests. This is a very difficult question: Is there ever good enough reason to take someone's life against their will, no matter how problematic their competence? This is just the sort of judgment that slippery slope adherents see as the beginning of medical murder.

52. The criteria are revised from originals in Prado 1990:173.

53. Battin 1984:297.

54. Quoted in Ayer and O'Grady 1992:197

55. Patients *themselves* may not be sure that they don't harbor some hope that they'll survive cessation of treatment. As in the cases of rationality and autonomy, we must work with reasonable degrees of understanding and intention. See Stanley 1992.

56. Requests for noninitiation of treatment also may be forms of assisted suicide or voluntary euthanasia, but it's unclear whether *doing nothing*, even if requested, can be assisting suicide.

57. To many health-care practitioners, as well as to many judges, refusal of treatment, requested cessation of treatment, or clinician-decided cessation of treatment isn't suicide or assisted suicide, because the underlying terminal condition is taken as the cause of death. This is lent credibility by the fact that we can never be certain that someone might not survive cessation of life-sustaining treatment.

58. "The judgment of a person who competently decides to commit suicide is . . . 'My expected future life, under the best conditions possible for me, is so bad that I judge it to be worse than no further continued life at all.' This seems to be . . . *exactly the same judgment* that some persons who decide to forego life-sustaining treatment make. The refusal of life-sustaining treatment is their means of ending their life; they intend to end their life because of its grim prospects. Their death now when they otherwise would not have died is self-inflicted, whether they take a lethal poison or disconnect a respirator" (Brock 1989:345; our emphasis). Note, though, that Brock glosses agency in saying "whether they take a lethal poison or disconnect a respirator." The point is that in most such cases, it isn't the patient that disconnects the respirator.

59. They may be paralyzed.

60. Starvation is an option, but even then patients must request not to be fed.

61. Competent patients may refuse treatment. Legal questions arise only when the patient in question isn't competent or is comatose and family members or surrogates want treatment stopped.

62. See Taylor 1995.

63. Euthanasia performed on a person in a coma would be neither voluntary nor involuntary; it would be nonvoluntary, meaning the concept of volition doesn't apply.

64. Whytehead and Chidwick 1980:29; our emphasis, the point of which is to call attention to the reconstrual of the preserving of life as the extension of the process of dying. "Prolonging dying" is a phrase that has fairly recently

gained widespread currency, and it has an undeniable intuitive clarity and appeal. Unfortunately, its currency may signal not better understanding but unreflective institutionalization of an unexamined idea through repetitive use. "Prolonging dying," as opposed to "prolonging life," makes it sound as if there is a clear difference, which is simply not the case, except in the most extreme cases. Believing that there is a clear difference here is dangerous, because of the elasticity of the notion of when dying begins.

65. Law Reform Commission of Canada 1983.

66. Narveson 1993:56.

67. When one agent is a clinician, with the status and power that that usually involves, and the other agent is a dependent patient, there is a danger that what appears to be assisted suicide is euthanasia.

68. Rorty claims that "there is no . . . criterion that we have not created in . . . creating a practice, no standard of rationality that is not an appeal to such a [practice-created] criterion" (Rorty 1982:xlii). Foucault worked to "isolat[e] the form of rationality presented as dominant, and endowed with the status of the one-and-only reason . . . to show that it is only one possible form among others" (Foucault 1988:27).

69. Even Rorty accepts this sense; in a letter regarding Prado 1990, he remarks that "rational" therein has "a quite definite sense, that used by those who claim that . . . suicide is always *ir*rational."

70. Battin 1982:301; our emphasis.

3

A GENUINE, UNIMPAIRED CHOICE

The idea that suicide isn't rational appears to be historically recent and is no doubt largely due to the impact of modern psychological and psychoanalytic theory.[1] Prior to about the second half of the nineteenth century, suicide was first and foremost thought to be *sinful*. The traditional philosophical debate on suicide focused on suicide's moral rightness or wrongness and, in doing so, took it for granted that suicide can be rational, at least in the sense of being a reasoned act knowingly and freely done. As we've noted, something can be a responsible act only if it is rational in this sense, and only responsible acts can be morally culpable. The traditional debate can be briefly characterized by contrasting Thomas Aquinas's and David Hume's articulations of the opposing positions that generate and sustain the debate. In his *Summa Theologica*, Aquinas argued that suicide is always wrong because it is against nature, because it injures the community, and because our lives are gifts of God and not ours to end.[2] This is the paradigm of the "life-as-gift" view, which casts being alive as entailing the responsibility to maintain one's own and others' lives. In his "On Suicide," Hume countered centuries of Thomistic thinking by arguing that suicide is permissible when it achieves greater value for the individual and society than does continuing to live.[3] This is the paradigm of the "life-as-possession" view, which casts remaining alive as falling within a person's discretion.

Despite hundreds of years of ongoing debate between adherents of the Thomistic and Humean positions on the morality of suicide, the prevalent contemporary view is that suicide isn't rational.[4] This idea is defended either on the basis that it is irrational and morally wrong to renounce the gift of life or on the basis that it is irrational to willingly relinquish life, even if doing so is not morally wrong. Supporting arguments range from philosophical contentions that suicide can't be coherently deliberated,[5] to psychological claims that we can't truly choose to die because we are incapable of understanding our own death,[6] to the popular view that self-destruction can only be a cowardly act of desperation.[7]

Regardless of the precise nature of the rejection of suicide, the point is that so long as it is judged to be anything less than a sensible choice in certain circumstances, assisting its commission can't be justified, since doing so would be compounding a wrong. Our task in this chapter is to show that suicide can be rational to the extent that it satisfies the requirements of our first criterion. This is necessary if we are to make our contention that suicide can be the best means to achieve the best purpose in some situations, and therefore may merit assistance in its commission. However, as will become clear, answering the question of how suicide can be judged rational according to the first criterion raises the even more daunting one of judging when the criterion's conditions are met.

THE UNIMPAIRMENT CRITERION

Our first criterion specifies that suicide, always assuming it to be an autonomous act, must be "a genuine option for the agent, chosen after deliberation consistent with accepted standards of reasoning and unimpaired by error, false beliefs, or lack of relevant information." We can clarify the first criterion by considering each of its two components: that suicide be *a genuine option*, and that suicide be chosen as a result of *sound, unimpaired deliberation.*[8]

Suicide's being a genuine option ironically has to do with its being what the American pragmatic philosopher William James called a "living" option.[9] James had in mind an option that a person finds it compelling to choose or reject, as opposed to merely understanding that it is a possible course of action. Given any situation, there are always numerous things one can do, but only a few of which one is actually moved to do. Suicide is the most drastic course of action open to anyone, and the genuine-option component of the first criterion requires that the abstract possibility of suicide become a compelling choice that someone feels moved to make decisively. Suicide can't be rational if its consideration remains abstract and, if committed, is done in an irresolute manner.[10]

The concern over the genuineness of suicide as an option also has to do with the autonomous nature of the act. Autonomy can be compromised in various ways. A common one is when the responsibility for what one does is shifted to another person or even an institution, as when an individual eases the burden of suicidal decision, and so erodes the genuineness of the option, by committing suicide under the "soothing moral shroud" discussed in the last chapter.[11] The genuineness component of our first criterion is designed to filter out cases like this to the extent possible, given the opacity of human motivation to both agents themselves and third parties.

We believe that suicide presents itself as a Jamesian living option, as something to be decisively done or not done, when an individual's interest in survival becomes problematic. Perhaps the most common way this happens is when survival is objectified by a terminal prognosis. One's very existence is pushed to conceptual arm's length by being diagnosed with a terminal condition or a chronic affliction of unbearable proportions.[12] When that occurs, a person may realize that worthwhile life and bare survival can be very different things. When survival is no longer of unquestionable worth and threatens to be actually disadvantageous, the interest in survival may be subordinated to other values, in particular, to the value put on quality of life. At that point there also may be recognition that one can choose not to live, that one can appropriate one's own inevitable death and avert needless misery. One may choose to live, but the choice of whether to live or die has become real in James's sense of being a living option.

A third aspect of the genuine-option component has to do with human adaptability and how even the most rational suicidal intention may change as time progresses. Even if at some point an individual decides to commit suicide rather than endure punishing survival, the weight given the quality of life will likely change as the prospect of death increases. What seemed intolerable earlier will probably begin to appear more benign. The initial decision to commit suicide may be weakened by familiarity with conditions that previously looked completely unacceptable.[13] Such weakening may mean that suicide ceases to be a genuine option; suicide may recede as a real choice and again become a mere abstract possibility. The rationality of its commission is then jeopardized.

Once suicide is a genuine option, once the abstract possibility becomes a concrete choice needing to be made, the question is how the person facing the option makes that choice. The second component of our criterion requires that the decision be made on the basis of sound reasoning about what best satisfies the individual's interests and values in the particular situation.

The nonimpairment component guards against suicide being an irrational act based on reasoning flawed by a breach of established standards. The most straightforward sort of impairment has to do with purely logical error, such as thinking that something follows from premises when it doesn't. For instance, it would not be rational to commit suicide after fallaciously concluding that because a parent had Alzheimer's disease, one will necessarily develop Alzheimer's.[14] A similar example, and one that is most pertinent here, is fallaciously concluding that because suicide is rationally permissible in a given situation, its commission is rationally required.[15]

Another sort of reasoning impairment has to do with what is taken as relevant to deliberation.[16] For instance, reasoning about commission of suicide would be impaired by taking a dream or an unsupported intuition as a relevant reason for killing oneself. A more problematic case would be if an individual claimed to hear supernatural voices advising suicide. Here we would begin to think of the impairment not as due to a particular lapse in reasoning but as due to an underlying pathological condition that would preclude rather than only test application of the criterion.

A still different sort of impairment is one in which a single idea or belief systematically distorts proper reasoning, but without being part of an underlying pathological condition. This could be an obsessive idea that, though not powerful enough to preclude rational deliberation, nonetheless skews reasoning. For instance, individuals might believe that, having fallen gravely ill, they don't deserve the cost and effort of care. Or someone might be unduly susceptible to the views of others. Innocent comments by a family member or a clinician about the cost of necessary care could constitute a highly detrimental influence on an overly impressionable person, for example, by causing a reason-impairing belief that one should commit suicide in order not to become a burden to others.

Even if a potential suicidist's reasoning is not flawed by procedural error, jeopardized by irrelevancies, or distorted by obsessive ideas, it still may not be sound because of false beliefs or lack of information. For instance, it would be irrational to commit suicide on the basis of a false belief that one had a terminal illness. Suicide would be equally irrational if committed while ignorant of some readily available fact, such as that a cure is available for a previously fatal disease.[17] The irrationality here would not be due to the ignorance itself but rather to lack of reasonable effort by the individual to learn or fully comprehend pertinent details about their condition. However, we aren't dealing in absolutes. Medicine is not an exact science; no prognosis is certain. Moreover, given relevant levels of expertise, it's hard to say what counts as sufficient effort on the part of a patient to acquire and check diagnostic and prognostic information. An individual might deliberate prudently and decide to commit suicide, and do so with good reason given the available data, but still do so on the basis of false belief or inadequate information. We can't demand more from those deliberating suicide than reasonable efforts to inform themselves about their situation and prospects. Our appeal to established reasoning standards must extend to established methods of acquiring and evaluating information. We have to accept that, in the absence of compelling evidence to the contrary, someone may decide to commit suicide on the basis of information that is by all usual standards adequate.[18]

It may be clear from the foregoing, but it merits explicit mention, that *rational* has two related but different contrasts. One is with *irrational* behavior, i.e., behavior based on flawed reasoning, compulsion, or derangement; the other is with *non-* or *arational* behavior, i.e., behavior that is unwitting, caused, or coerced.[19] Our primary concern is with the claim that suicide is irrational; we are only indirectly concerned with nonrational or arational behavior. Our aim is to show that the decision to end one's own life may be the outcome of sane, prudent, judicious deliberation about a choice that presents itself forcibly to an individual in a critical situation.

The points made about the genuineness of suicide as an option and nonimpairment of reasoning have a common thread running through them, which is the pivotal importance of the role of others in suicidal deliberation. Caregivers, family members, and friends play a crucial role in assessing reasoning and motivation in suicidal deliberation and in providing necessary information. Our first criterion's purpose is to ensure that when suicide is chosen as a course of action, it is an autonomous choice based on sound reasoning. But people have no reliable way of assessing their own motives and reasoning about emotionally charged matters. Not only that, but as we noted earlier, human actions "are never wholly free from emotion, training, circumstantial coercion, or other arational components."[20] There are certainly emotional factors and circumstantial coercion in suicidal deliberation, and they may impair reasoning in ways no single individual can detect and correct. Other people, with different and more objective perspectives, can better judge whether unrealistic optimism or morbid pessimism is seriously distorting someone's appraisal of a critical situation. At the very least, a variety of construals of that situation provides an individual with a means to gain some distance from their initial and perhaps skewed assessment. This advantage relates to what may be the most familiar contribution others make to the assessment of a grievous personal crisis, which is to afford opportunities to air fears that often become more manageable in being voiced. A person considering suicide also needs authoritative information. Committing suicide for medical reasons is basically a matter of trading time left for avoidance of what that time will bring, so the factual basis for suicidal deliberation must be as solid as possible. No single individual can hope to have the expertise and information to ensure that it is.

MEETING THE REQUIREMENT

With an understanding of the genuineness and nonimpairment components of our first criterion, we can consider the difficult matter of judging when the first criterion's requirements are met. The genuineness and nonimpairment conditions require that those considering suicide do so autonomously and on the basis of sound reasoning. Someone considering whether to assist suicide must assess whether the potential suicidist is choosing to die autonomously and on the basis of sound reasoning. If that is not the case, then assisting suicide is to wrongly facilitate an irrational self-destructive act, which is never justified. We should note, though, that although suicide and assisted suicide are ruled out if the first criterion's requirements aren't met, some form of euthanasia may be acceptable for humane reasons.

In ideal situations, dialogue among several concerned individuals and the potential suicidist enables effective assessment and sound judgment about whether the first criterion's conditions are met. But questions arise about the focus of assessment in cases of assisted suicide in medical contexts, and these questions mark a major though hard to articulate conflict between theory and practice.

The conflict is due to how clinicians' assessments of requests for assisted suicide tend to be carried out in terms of holistic assessment of patients. This means not only that patients' medical conditions and prognoses are integral and important parts of those assessments but also that they may overshadow patients' reasoning and wishes. Against this, theoreticians see it as dangerous to so broaden the scope of assessment, because other factors may obscure or outweigh confused reasoning. On the one hand, reliance on holistic assessment means that decisions about whether or not to assist suicide are better grounded and informed than they otherwise might be; on the other hand, it means that such considerations as very poor prognoses might unduly prevail over patients' confusions or ambivalences. For theoreticians and clinicians, the question is basically about the relative priority given to patients' reasoning about self-destruction as opposed to their overall states of mind and medical conditions.

What makes the assessment-focus conflict hard to articulate is the difficulty of distinguishing the two approaches without caricaturing clinicians as blind to the forest and theoreticians as blind to the trees. We can best proceed by focusing on something in particular that generates opposing positions representative of the two approaches. In our own collaboration, we found ourselves on opposite sides of the assessment-focus conflict because of our disagreement on the significance of belief in an afterlife to the rationality of suicide. The ubiquity of the belief is undeniable,[21] so we agree that it poses a real issue, but while one of us sees the belief's significance as considerable when the focus of assessment is suicidal deliberation, the other sees it as negligible when the focus is the potential suicidist's general state. Consideration of the belief's perceived significance helps clarify the assessment-focus conflict.

Strictly interpreted, our first criterion counts belief in an afterlife as an impairment to rational suicide to the extent that the belief obscures the finality of death. However, it is most important to understand that the problem is not the rationality of the belief itself. Our appeal regarding rationality is to established standards of reasoning, and those standards allow belief in an afterlife. Having the belief is the rule in our culture, and it is supported by the major religions and their most respected theologians. There is also no scarcity of secular philosophers and scientists who defend belief in an afterlife. These people and institutions contribute to defining our culture and so are in part responsible for setting and administering our established standards of reasoning. It would be illegitimate to appeal to established standards regarding assessment of the soundness of suicidal deliberation but to exclude a particular belief that those standards allow.[22] Nor is the problem the factual question of the truth or falsity of the belief, since it is impossible to establish either conclusively. The problem is whether having the belief impairs suicidal reasoning by interpreting death as not an end but a new beginning. On a strict interpretation of the first criterion, even if belief in an afterlife is rational, its possession blunts vivid awareness of the consequences of suicide and so jeopardizes its rationality. On a contextual and empathic interpretation of the first criterion, since the belief is rational, it has no special significance for the rationality of suicidal deliberation.

To better explain the problem posed by belief in an afterlife, consider that though the contemporary view that suicide is irrational is wrongheaded, it does appeal to an obvious fact: Life is irretrievable once lost.[23] Because of this hard fact, in assessing whether one would be better off dying than living through something awful, the finality of death has to be weighed against another hard fact: There can be no certainty that what is avoided by dying might not be tolerable or be alleviated by compensating value.[24] It would seem, then, that choosing to die, even in dire circumstances, could always be precipitous, and thus always less than rational. This is the core practical—i.e., nonmoral—reason for not accepting suicide as rational: Given our limited knowledge, ending one's own life doesn't make the best sense, because our expectations about our future are never sure enough to justify forgoing that future.

What emerges is that underlying the rejection of suicide as irrational because of the finality of death is the conception of death as personal annihilation. Only if death *is* annihilation is it always better to take one's chances living rather than dying to avoid something. The force of the point is that no one can rationally prefer total nonexistence to even punishing existence.[25] Given the assumption that death is annihilation, it does seem irrational to willingly forfeit life unless it is certain that it has become both totally unbearable and utterly hopeless with respect to any chance of betterment.

The problem posed by thinking that death isn't personal annihilation, the belief in an afterlife, is that if death is believed to be some sort of transition to another level of existence, consideration of suicide is very different than if death is believed to be the absolute end of personal existence. Death retains its force, but it would be naïve to deny that it is one thing to contemplate ending your life if you think that that would be the end of your existence and quite another thing to contemplate ending your "earthly" life with some confidence that you will continue in another realm. It can be argued that this difference is basically immaterial to assessing the rationality of suicide, because of the cultural acceptability and ubiquity of belief in an afterlife. However, it also can be argued that belief in an afterlife is an impairment to suicidal reasoning, not because the belief is itself irrational but because it blunts vivid awareness of suicide's consequences.

For many theoreticians, belief in an afterlife jeopardizes suicidal deliberation because of its likely dulling effect on awareness and intention of consequences. Belief in an afterlife by the person lending assistance also may jeopardize the permissibility of assisted suicide by seeming to reduce the gravity of suicide. Death is seen not as the termination of existence but as a transition to another form of existence, so assisting suicide isn't considered participation in self-annihilation. Moreover, the reduction affects the moral gravity of suicide and assisted suicide as well, because ending one's own life, or helping others to end their lives, isn't seen as annihilating oneself or helping others annihilate themselves. The theoretical view, then, is that because of its gravity, suicide and assisted suicide should be deliberated on the basis of a worst-case scenario—i.e., on the assumption that death is annihilation. The rationale is that since suicide is an irrevocable act, and since there is no reliable evidence that there is an afterlife, suicide must be deliberated on the assumption that self-destruction is just that. This is not to say that belief in an afterlife precludes sound suicidal deliberation outright; it is to say that the possibility that death is personal annihilation must be seriously acknowledged and allowed for in the making of a decision to end one's life.

For most clinicians and many clinical ethicists, belief in an afterlife doesn't play a significant role in justifying suicide and assisted suicide. For one thing, the patient requesting assisted suicide may hold the belief but still understand that it's only a belief and not certain knowledge. If not, if the belief is held in some obsessive way that raises serious questions for clinicians, it most likely will be part of a more general problematic condition that would preclude assisted suicide by raising questions about competence. More important is that requests for assisted suicide are usually made in the context of great suffering and stress, and most often in hopeless situations. In such circumstances, belief in an afterlife simply doesn't seem significant; it appears to play no real part in patients not wanting to live on in punishing circumstances.

Reference to circumstances brings us back to the matter of the focus of assessment in the evaluation of requests for assisted suicide. If we're looking first at a potential suicidist's chain of reasoning, as most theoreticians think we should, we might find that reasoning flawed by belief in an afterlife. But if we're looking first at patients' circumstances, belief in an afterlife may be immaterial. In assessing requests for assisted suicide, clinicians rarely attempt to evaluate a patient's particular reasoning. They don't proceed as a theoretician would, by tracing the logical sequence of the deliberation and testing the cogency of reasons for acting in one or way another. Clinicians need to evaluate *the patient*, in the sense of holistically evaluating the individual as either generally competent or not.

Occasions for evaluating patient competence are usually specific treatment decisions, but before asking for a patient's consent to a particular surgical procedure, for instance, clinicians must assess whether the patient is competent to make responsible decisions, or whether the required decision must be relegated to a surrogate decision maker.[26] Clinicians' assessments, though keyed to specific decisions, have to begin with such considerations as whether a patient is better able to make decisions at a particular time of day, before or after medication, or simply when having a "good day" in the case of early dementia patients. The object of assessment, then, is the patient, not a particular line of reasoning conducted by the patient. Clinicians evaluate patients' understanding of assisted suicide just as they do patients' understanding of other treatment options: They begin with the patient's general competence, and rightly so, because that competence is problematic in medical situations for reasons ranging from the effects of stress and medication to clinical depression and dementia.

Theoreticians take general competence to make rational decisions as given; their assessment of reasoning is more or less context-free. What they consider is formulation of premises and inferential progression to a conclusion. They test that progression for consistency and validity and, to the extent possible, test the truth of the premises to determine the soundness of the reasoning.[27] If the reasoning is sound, then the conclusion is taken as established. The assessment process is no different because the premises and conclusion happen to be about self-destruction. Clinicians weigh requests for assisted suicide against patients' conditions, prospects, and competence, rather than against patients' specific deliberations about the relative advantages of living or dying. Clinicians' main concern is patients' capacity to make responsible decisions, not the logical mechanics of patients' progress from premises to conclusions in making their decisions. Given that the patients they deal with are under great pressure and vulnerable to all sorts of influences, the key question is whether those patients *can* make sound, informed decisions.

Clinicians' first concern in assessing requests for assisted suicide is to eliminate preclusive incapacity due to underlying conditions such as clinical depression. Therefore, impairment of the sort our first criterion addresses is initially dealt with by judging patients' competence. Whether a patient is able to reason clearly isn't further tested by evaluating the formulating of premises, the drawing of inferences, and the reaching of valid conclusions.[28] If patients are judged competent, it tends to be assumed that their reasoning isn't significantly impaired. Since patients' reasoning about relinquishing life is not assessed in isolation,[29] expression of one or another problematic belief usually is seen as significant only if it is thought to be symptomatic of serious instability. For instance, if a patient were to voice paranoid delusions about their illness being due to a political conspiracy, that patient's request for assisted suicide likely would be ignored or at most communicated to a family member or other surrogate decision maker. But if in the process of requesting assisted suicide a patient mentioned hoping "to go to heaven," for example, that would have little or no effect on clinicians' assessment of competence.

Initially, holistic assessment of patients' competence looks considerably more realistic than assessment of their suicidal reasoning. But if theoreticians' preferred detailed assessment may be vitiated by crucial contextual considerations, clinicians' broader assessments are prey to the weight consciously or unconsciously but invariably given the patient's medical condition, as well as to a myriad of institutional and personal influences.[30] The assessment-focus question, then, isn't as straightforward as it looks, regardless of how easy it may be to make the theoretical look pedantically obtrusive to caring treatment.

The kinds of questions that shape holistic assessment of patients who request assisted suicide—or voluntary euthanasia—are of this sort:[31] (1) How stable is the request; does it appear to result from long-term consideration or only short-term reaction to a terminal prognosis; are there frequent changes of mind about the request? (2) Does the request mask anything; is it prompted by clinical depression or perhaps by some depressive side effect of medication? (3) Is the request an attempt to shift the burden of a difficult decision?[32] (4) How accurate are the patient's nonmedical claims regarding family attitudes and the like? (5) Has there been frank discussion with loved ones; has the patient considered the effect of suicide on others? (6) Is the request driven by fear of becoming a burden? (7) Is the patient possibly being manipulated by family members? These questions are complemented by more medically focused ones: (8) Is the point of the request to end present intractable pain or to avoid expected pain? (9) Is the medical condition prompting the request adequately understood by the patient? (10) Does the pain appear to be punishing enough to merit dying to relieve it? How reliable is the prognosis? (11) Will continued treatment alter the prognosis in a significant way and thus offer the patient hope, or will further treatment merely prolong dying? (12) Can the patient's request be met simply by cessation of treatment, or would more intrusive measures be necessary?

Only the first two of these dozen typical questions have to do directly with the potential suicidist's reasoning.[33] Even then, the questions are about stability and possible underlying problems, not about clear as opposed to confused reasoning. A patient could be quite persistent over time about a request for assisted suicide and not be clinically depressed, yet still be reasoning in a confused manner—for instance, taking it as given that, unlike others, they don't merit protracted and costly terminal care. But the more worrying point is the likelihood that if the answers to the other ten questions are of the right sort, problematic answers to the first two will be heavily discounted or ignored. Moreover, problematic answers to the first two questions may not be recognized as problematic if the focus is not on deliberation but on general competence. A patient's expressed expectations about an afterlife may appear mundane, but they could conceal deep confusion. For instance, if someone requests assisted suicide in order to rejoin a long-dead spouse, the fact that they are in a terminal condition may make a clinician accede to the request for the wrong reasons. The patient's medical condition shouldn't override the fact that killing oneself because of a conviction that death is a transition to a happier version of past life isn't rational. Suicidal deliberation, to be rational, must include consideration that one may utterly cease to exist on dying.[34]

Admittedly, it is difficult to assess the role and importance of individual beliefs. For instance, expression of belief in an afterlife could be no more impairing than metaphorical recognition of an illusion we use to cope with our mortality. The expression may play a self-consoling role rather than indicate a problem with deliberation. In contrast, an individual who denies belief in an afterlife, or expresses only the most innocuous hopes about the heaven that religion promises, actually may have reason-impairing ideas about the nature of death.[35] Certainly neither clinicians nor even clinical ethicists can be expected to conduct extensive philosophical and theological analyses in evaluating patients' requests for assisted suicide. Additionally, ordinary people unschooled in rigorous abstract reasoning are unlikely to be capable of articulating precisely what it is they believe about the nature of death and how what they believe figures in their suicidal deliberation.[36]

Is assessment of suicidal deliberation simply impractical, and must we be satisfied with assessment of general competence? Some believe that this is the case and that sound decisions to end life or to help patients end their lives are regularly and rightly made in clinical practice on the basis of assessment of competence. The trouble is that what may well be presently adequate clinical practice regarding assisted suicide could prove inadequate if assisted suicide becomes an accepted convention. The very fact of assisted suicide becoming a conventional option may change its practice for the worse.[37] For instance, if dire prognoses currently prompt clinicians to occasionally ignore patients' flawed suicidal reasoning, those same prognoses could prompt systematic indifference to patient confusion when requests for assisted suicide multiply. There is a need to ensure that institutionalization of present practices, both as conducted in hospitals and as taught in medical schools, won't devolve into a mess that some future generation will have to set right. The necessity is to practice assisted suicide—and voluntary euthanasia—in a way that doesn't degenerate into *routine*. As Sandel puts it, we need to find a way to provide assistance in the commission of suicide that *"preserves the moral burden of hastening death."*[38]

Possible deterioration of clinical practices regarding assisted suicide basically has to do with how seriously we take death and how far we are prepared to go to ensure that someone choosing to die is doing the right thing, both in their view and in ours. The present widespread illegality of assisted suicide guarantees that careful thought is given to contravening prohibitions, so helping someone to die is taken quite seriously—if only for fear of repercussions. But with the prohibitions removed, we simply don't know how attitudes may change. Many agree with Seneca's observation that there are times when we should relinquish life for reasons "not as pressing as they might be," because the reasons that restrain us are "not so pressing either."[39] Those same people think that if there are good medical reasons for people to relinquish life, we ought not to probe their own reasons too deeply and comply with their reasonable requests for aid in dying. There are others who, even though advocates of assisted suicide, believe that "[a] terminally ill patient should be helped to die only after every alternative has been exhausted."[40] Their view is that we must be continuously on guard against taking self-inflicted death too lightly and allowing ourselves to disdain "life that is dependent."[41]

With respect to possibly confused reasoning, it may be that in evaluating requests for assisted suicide, nothing more can practically be done than to put the question of death's possibly annihilatory nature to patients making the requests.[42] This is usually difficult and sometimes may even be somewhat cruel, but it needs to be done, regardless of the vulnerability and precariousness of suffering patients' states of mind.[43] The implication here is that holistic assessment of patients requesting assisted suicide is the more practically viable approach in medical contexts, and that more narrowly focused assessment of reasoning has to be left to clinicians' discretion as to when it's needed and the extent to which it should be pursued.[44] In the majority of cases, it is enough if patients respond inappropriately to discussions of their requests for assisted suicide. If clinicians' efforts to discuss the seriousness of the requests elicit irrational responses, such as complete refusal to enter into discussion or angry denouncement of prying, those responses themselves suffice to raise questions about patients' competence to make life-or-death decisions. Given seriously inappropriate responses, especially persistent ones, there is no need to sift through problematic beliefs.

A DOSE OF REALITY

Despite the fact that it looks as if their present holistic assessment practice edges out a more focused assessment of reasoning, a great deal of the foregoing will strike many clinicians as quite pointless. They will be inclined to write it off as so much more abstract theorizing having little to do with what they face on a daily basis. When a patient is in agony and repeatedly asks or even begs to be helped to die, questions about whether the patient's desire to die is based on sound reasoning may look almost comic in their irrelevance. In any case, how could we ever determine, without lengthy philosophical discussion and no small amount of psychoanalysis, just what someone believes and how their beliefs operate in their suicidal deliberation? And does it matter, for instance, what afterlife beliefs someone may have, so long as they understand that suicide will end their *earthly* life? It's certainly arguable that such factors as belief in an afterlife simply aren't material to decisions about assisting the suicides of patients whose lives are all but over and have ceased to be a blessing and have become a punishing, destructive curse. When our strongest painkillers make little difference, except that enough of them will kill, it's hard to take seriously the idea that a suffering individual may want to die for shaky intellectual reasons or should be kept alive long enough to discuss in depth just why they want to die.

However, although these sentiments are certainly forceful, they miss the point. What matters most here is how clinicians conceive of assisting suicide, and that's determined as much by training as by practical experience. The balance between theoretical requirements and practical demands that we are trying to facilitate has to be first achieved not in a cancer ward or an intensive care unit but in the training of clinicians. It is only then that balance may be achieved at the bedside. What is at issue is how clinicians approach and construe situations in which they have to deal with people who are dying far too slowly for their own good. The considerations we've discussed about nonimpairment and genuineness aren't a laundry list to be run through while dealing with patients; they are considerations that should become second nature for properly trained clinicians who must deal with people who request assisted suicide. Probing to determine whether a suicidal impulse is a product of sound or impaired reasoning should be automatic to a clinician who has to assess such requests.

Of course, many clinicians hotly maintain that such probing is done now, and they are right, up to a point. But as alluded to before, the question isn't really about what good clinicians do *now*; the question is what will happen if assisted suicide becomes a conventional treatment option. We must do everything we can to prevent such things as terminal prognoses from overshadowing people. If it's currently unacceptable for a man or woman to become "the gallbladder in 214," it's still more unacceptable for a terminally ill woman or man considering suicide to become the "better-off-dead in 214." One important way to prevent that is to greatly intensify present efforts to mold clinicians to be concerned first with terminal patients' thinking, with what makes those patients *persons*, and only second with their medical conditions and prospects.

Probing a potential suicidist's reasoning needn't be an exercise in logic. Basically, it's a matter of recognizing that someone requesting assisted suicide is one of *us* and thus vulnerable to fear, confusion, intimidation, and all the other things that can make people do things they really aren't ready to do or perhaps don't even want to do. For the sake of our own humanity, we can't let others' decisions to die become so many more decisions about the productivity of treatment or its lack. Our first criterion requires that even the most harried and pressed clinician make the time to probe a patient's decision to die,[45] but that doesn't mean temporarily abandoning the clinician's role and adopting that of the logician. It means resisting the momentum of routine and listening carefully to whether another human being is making sense about wanting to cease to live.[46]

The problem posed by the first criterion's nonimpairment requirement in medical contexts comes to this: Clinicians making decisions about whether or not to accede to requests for assisted suicide are trained to base their procedural decisions on patients' general competence, medical conditions, and prognoses. These are, after all, the aspects of patients' situations that concern them professionally. When other considerations are weighed, they tend to be such things as family members' acceptance of treatment decisions, legal responsibilities, and the like. Potential suicidists' reasoning normally isn't probed in any depth, being evaluated mostly for indications of underlying clinical depression, psychopathology, and so forth. If patients are judged competent to make decisions about their own treatment or its cessation, their reasoning is assumed to be sound. This is in part because clinicians generally lack the training to engage in fine-grained analysis of reasoning, and in part because once patients are judged competent, many clinicians see no cause to be suspicious of their reasoning. The danger, then, is basically that patients may be assisted in suicide despite counterindications lying below the surface. The most relevant counterindications here are confusion and avoidance of adequate recognition of consequences.

For theoreticians, the nonimpairment requirement of the first criterion calls for more than present clinical assessment practices include, even if only in anticipation of assisted suicide becoming a conventional option. The "more" is finer-grained analysis of suicidal deliberation in evaluation of requests for assisted suicide. But theoreticians and clinical ethicists concede the practical difficulties of finer-grained analysis, as well as that the overly strict interpretation of the nonimpairment requirement could prevent as many warranted assisted suicides as are now prevented by illegality.

An obvious way to achieve a compromise, and so a balance of theoretical and clinical requirements, is to have more careful probing of suicidal deliberation within the boundaries of current holistic assessment of patient competence. However, this compromise isn't something that can be achieved by issuing still more guidelines to overregulated clinicians. The compromise can be achieved only by longer-term changes in clinicians' training. Just as medical ethics is being recognized as an essential part of medical training, instruction in more thorough appraisal of reasoning must be recognized as equally essential. But this is easily said; the hard part is knowing how to bring it about. Tacking on a course in informal logic to the medical curriculum, although advisable,[47] won't do the job. The challenge is to better understand and direct how clinicians-in-training adopt their professional values and priorities.

The crucial point is that deciding whether a request for assisted suicide should be acceded to requires determining whether suicide is rational for the individual in question. That assessment clearly includes the individual's medical condition and prospects, but those factors mustn't be taken as decisive. In other words, the process of appraising a request for assisted suicide is two-pronged: One prong has to do with the patient's medical circumstances, the other with the patient's reasoning.

If the latter is somehow flawed, some other form of aid in dying may be justified, but not assisted *suicide*. Another way of putting the point is that appraising a request for assisted suicide requires recognizing and allowing for a patient's humanity and the ambivalences and confusions it entails, as well as attending to what's on the patient's chart. The tough question is what to do about cases in which there is a significant gap between good medical reasons for an individual to relinquish life and that individual's own reasons for wanting to do so.

The first criterion attempts to ensure that an individual's decision to relinquish life is sound by establishing that suicide is a genuine, unimpaired choice for and by that individual, and that self-destruction best serves that individual's values and interests. The trouble starts when someone who would be best off not living, to avoid predictable unnecessary suffering, chooses not to live but does so on the basis of confused reasoning. Confused reasoning renders the resulting decision to commit suicide not rational or at least not fully rational. Suicide in the particular case, then, is *not* the best means to achieve the best purpose. For example, as we considered earlier, the individual may choose to commit suicide while totally convinced that death isn't an end but a transition to a new life. Whatever its actual merits, this belief, *if unquestioned*, masks the possibly annihilatory consequences of self-destruction, so the suicidist may relinquish life absolutely without intending to do so. This sort of decision-vitiating confusion may not be a problem for the *suicidist*, but what makes it crucial for us is that our concern here is *assisted* suicide. Those assisting suicide done on the basis of confused reasoning share the responsibility for an irrational—or at least partly irrational—self-destructive act. What application of the first criterion comes to, then, is protection for those assisting suicide. Just as following regulations is protection against negative legal repercussions, applying the first criterion is protection against compounding irrational behavior, and that is ultimately protection against inhumanity.

However, whether suicide is or isn't rational in being a genuine, unimpaired option is not the end of the matter. Even if suicide is rational, in the sense that the decision is reached in a sound manner according to the first criterion, questions remain about values and interests. In the next chapter we turn to the matter of motivating values.

SUMMARY

Our first criterion applies to suicidal decisions that are made freely, resolutely, and knowingly. The criterion requires that to be rational, suicide must present itself as a real option, and the reasoning leading to the suicidal decision must be unimpaired. Making a rational decision to commit suicide may be jeopardized by confusion, error, and/or ignorance, so it's crucial that the potential suicidist have the discursive support of friends and caregivers to ensure that the decision made is as balanced and informed as possible. Only if suicide is rational is it permissible to assist its commission. Assisted suicide in medical contexts raises the question of clinicians' focus of assessment in appraising requests for assisted suicide. The first criterion calls for the focus of assessment to be the potential suicidist's reasoning, but in medical contexts, the indicated focus of assessment is patient competence in light of medical conditions and prognoses. This raises the special problem that flawed or confused suicidal reasoning may be ignored or overridden for medical reasons that independently show suicide to best serve a patient's interests. Additionally, in clinical settings, there are practical obstacles to assessment of reasoning being pressed much beyond the level at which patients are judged competent to make major treatment decisions. It seems there may be little option but to accept patients' reasoning at face value if there is no compelling cause to suspect incompetence. Nonetheless, there is room to approach more closely the theoretical requirement that reasoning be closely assessed. This may be done by ensuring that medical training inculcates greater sensitivity to the importance of unimpaired reasoning. The objective is to achieve a better balance, in clinicians' practices, between appraising requests for assisted suicide on the basis of medical particulars and establishing that patients are choosing to relinquish their lives on the basis of sound reasoning.

NOTES

1. Not only did those theories provide accounts of suicide as pathological, they also provided the vocabulary and the apparent authority for articulation of the conventional negative attitude toward suicide.

2. See Honderich 1995:859. Aquinas's third claim together with the commandment not to kill grounds Catholic prohibition of suicide. The commandment is read by other faiths as including oneself. See Exodus 20:1–17 and Deuteronomy 5:6–21. The common view is that, as a gift of God, life isn't ours to take.

3. Hume [1776] 1826.

4. Again, this is taken as "an article of commonsensism" (Donnelly 1978:89; see Roy, Williams, and Dickens 1994:412).

5. E.g., the "incommensurability" or "lack of contrast" argument, which holds that since being dead is an unknown and unknowable nonstate, it is incoherent to try to evaluate being dead in suicidal deliberation. The argument's main premise is that "the opacity of death and its consequent incommensurability with life" make it impossible to judge "that a person is better off dead" (Audi 1995:252). The reference is to euthanasia, but the point applies equally to suicide.

If we can't evaluate the relative merits of life and death, then suicidal deliberation is a sham, and any self-destructive behavior it leads to will be a product of confusion. To account for counterexamples in which we would judge self-destruction to be the only sensible choice, as in cases of surcease suicide, those who endorse the incommensurability argument redefine suicide to exclude self-inflicted death in utterly hopeless situations. Self-destruction is tolerated when a person is in horrendous and irreparable agony, when the inescapable alternative to dying is committing a gross moral wrong, and as a heroic sacrifice for the good of others. According to those who endorse this argument, self-destruction in these cases is not considered suicide.

What is needed to defeat the incommensurability argument is not a counterargument but clarification of its own premises. The argument's basic error is that being dead is not one of the evaluated alternatives in suicidal deliberation. The alternatives considered in suicidal deliberation are not being alive and being dead; the alternatives that are deliberated are whether to endure a certain condition or not to endure it, when the only way to escape it is to die. The incommensurability argument works only if suicidal deliberation is wrongly construed as an attempt to evaluate being dead against being alive. Once that is appreciated, the rationality of suicide is not precluded by death being an unknown and unknowable nonstate.

6. See Battin 1984:299. We think that this claim is simply too vague to consider, and again, in "the absence of any compelling evidence to the contrary," we have to accept that someone may choose to die "on the basis of reasoning which is by all usual standards adequate" (Battin 1984:301).

7. It is interesting how suicide is often described as "the easy way out," as if there were a deep obligation to endure whatever excruciating pain might befall one. See Hamel and DuBose 1996; Hentoff 1996.

8. *Sound* commonly means "cogent" and "sensible." We use *sound* in this sense, but with the added technical sense in which an argument is sound when

its premises are true and its conclusion is valid, i.e., it follows logically from the premises.

9. James was concerned with religious faith as a "living" option that couldn't be ignored (James 1897:2–4).

10. Sometimes people experiment with "going through the motions," perhaps to test their own resolve, and suddenly act on impulse. One of us was instrumental in a despondent student's being committed for a five-day psychiatric observation after she nearly hanged herself while trying out "how it felt" to go about killing herself. Though she claimed that she did not intend to, at some point she stepped off whatever she was standing on. She was not killed only because the rope's support gave way. Suicide committed in this manner is not a rational act.

11. Kristol 1993. Note that while shifting responsibility may mean that an act is not rational as suicide, that does not preclude it from being rational as euthanasia if, in fact, another assumes responsibility for the death of the person in question.

12. Alzheimer's disease, for instance, is not itself a terminal illness, in the sense that one may live for many years before brain deterioration proves fatal and would likely die of some other cause well before that point.

13. In a clinic that one of us is aware of, patients who are terminally ill are often provided with enough medication to painlessly commit suicide if they choose. Their diseases have symptoms that cause severe pain and suffering, and at the time of diagnosis, it is common to hear talk of suicide. But as the disease progresses, talk of suicide tends to give way to acceptance of symptoms that at the outset were thought intolerable. As far as we've determined, none of these patients has actually committed suicide.

14. There is strong evidence that a disposition to develop Alzheimer's is genetic, but the likelihood that a given individual will develop the disease varies, depending on whether one or both parents developed the disease, and is in any case not certain.

15. There is nothing illogical about understanding that one would be better off dying than enduring something and choosing not to die. It may be foolish, but it isn't incoherent.

16. For instance; the appearance of the Hale-Bopp comet in March and April of 1997 was taken by the Heaven's Gate cult members as a sign that they should commit suicide. See Bruni 1997.

17. This is not to suggest that a clinician might fail to inform a patient about an available cure, but that a patient may make little or no effort to understand what they are told after the initial devastating diagnosis.

18. Here we paraphrase Battin 1984:301.

19. Recall that if suicide is a deranged act or a caused behavior, it isn't rational, so it isn't immoral either. One is not culpable for behavior that is caused or deranged. Note that here we are not commenting on whether such a suicide might not be *reasonable* from both first- and third-person perspectives.

20. Battin 1984:297

21. In informal discussions with five hospital chaplains, one of us found that in all their combined years of practice, only one chaplain, and only once, had talked with a dying individual who did not speak of an afterlife.

22. One may call into question the rationality of a particular cultural belief system on the grounds that it incorporates false beliefs, but the rationality of the individual members of that culture who hold those beliefs can't be impugned simply because they hold their culture's prevalent beliefs. See Battin 1982:302. If one wants to impugn the rationality of an individual in a particular culture that incorporates false beliefs, it must be established that the individual should know better. In the case of belief in an afterlife, neither side has reliable grounds on which to claim that someone should know better, since there is no conclusive evidence for or against the truth of the belief.

23. Not even those faiths that include belief in reincarnation hold that what follows death is a continuation of the same life.

24. This is Battin's point that in considering suicide as an alternative to suffering, we have to look at "the amount of other experience permitted . . . and whether this other experience is of intrinsic value" (Battin 1984:312).

25. This is the essence of the incommensurability argument: Nonexistence can't be valued over even the worst sort of existence, because as a nonstate it can't coherently be evaluatively compared with existing.

26. But see Hardwig 1993.

27. An argument with false premises may be *valid* but not *sound*.

28. The questions used in initiating assessment of a patient's competence have to do with knowing the day of the week or who heads the government, not with violation of *modes ponens*.

29. Aside from considering patients' medical conditions and prognoses, attending clinicians form educated impressions of their patients. Some patients are quite matter-of-fact about their situations, others are despondent, and still others experience wide mood swings. Awareness of such things contributes to how clinicians take what their patients say.

30. Schneiderman et al. 1993 ; see also Hardwig 1993.

31. Though we've added one or two, here we mainly paraphrase some of seventeen questions listed by Battin (1994:272–5) as appropriate to assessing requests for assisted suicide.

32. Recall the "soothing moral shroud" point (Kristol 1993).

33. Though the third appears to be about reasoning, it's really a psychological question about something like self-deception.

34. Compare Battin 1984:299.

35. One of us had a student in a philosophy of religion class who believed that there was no spiritual afterlife but that after death we're reincarnated as strangers to keep track of loved ones.

36. A typical situation in which these obstacles are evident is when a hastened death is in fact in a patient's best interests, and the patient consistently

expresses a wish to die, but that wish is simply repeated and probing questions are ignored, possibly for lack of understanding.

37. Sandel 1997:27; Steinfels 1997a.

38. Sandel 1997:27.

39. Seneca (1969) tells us that "[T]here are . . . occasions on which a man should leave life . . . for reasons . . . not as pressing as they might be—the reasons which restrain us being not so pressing either."

40. Quill and Rollin 1996. Note that "every alternative" here is not a hopeless catchall and refers to relevant medical treatment alternatives for particular conditions.

41. Steinfels 1997a: 12.

42. Note that if the patients in question are competent enough to request aid in dying, they are competent enough to be asked if they understand what they are requesting. The questions put here are of the same order as those put to patients asked to provide "informed consent" regarding surgical procedures. The point is not to raise philosophical issues about death but to establish that the patients appreciate what they are requesting. The issue of the capacity for autonomous decisions obviously arises here, but as we said before, we have to work with what is possible in the circumstances, not absolutes.

43. Clearly, if a patient is too overwrought, then the request for aid in dying must be referred to the next of kin or surrogate decision makers.

44. If an attending clinician judges that a patient requesting assisted suicide hasn't adequately considered some aspect of their decision, whether it be that death is the end of existence or that the patient's terminal prognosis is still inconclusive, the clinician faces a judgment call on how to proceed. But the question then is really about the competence of the patient, not about a particular bit of reasoning on their part.

45. Nor is it enough to use some pat formula in a condescending manner designed to reassure. The effort must be genuine and not a patronizing exercise.

46. It may well be that a patient's decision is ill founded, that assisted suicide is not permissible, and that it is still best for the patient in question to die. If that is the case, then clinicians may need to accept the responsibility of performing some form of euthanasia. The corollary is that society must assume the burden of sanctioning euthanasia rather than just legalizing assisted suicide and then not looking too closely at the reasons for it. Australia has done this. See "Australian Man First in World to Die with Legal Euthanasia," *New York Times*, September 26, 1996.

47. A recent study found that more than 33 percent of tested residents accepted logical fallacies of relevance in descriptions of cases, more than 25 percent accepted logical fallacies of induction, and a surprising *64 percent* accepted circular reasoning. Just over 20 percent accepted false premises. The implication is that residents were considerably more secure in medical knowledge than in reasoning applying that knowledge. Auclair et al. 1996:102.

4

ACCESSIBLE MOTIVATION

The second criterion for rational suicide requires that "the agent's motivating values[1] are cogent to others, not unduly contravening the agent's interests." To be rational, suicide must be motivated by values or priorities that pass the test of peer assessment by being found cogent, if not compelling, by others. This means that others must judge that the agent's motivating values or priorities, the reasons for committing suicide, make good enough sense to warrant self-destruction and override the suicidist's basic interest in continued life.

The criterion's primary role is to ensure that the reasons why someone chooses to relinquish life are reasonable ones and would motivate others to take their lives in the same circumstances.[2] This doesn't just mean that the motives for committing suicide have to be understandable, as Choron seems to think is enough; it means that they have to be accepted as convincing reasons for self-destruction. The criterion is concerned with motivating values or priorities that might appear perfectly reasonable to someone at a particular time, but only because their judgment is distorted by confused reasoning, despondency, or serious emotional upset.[3] Others would find such motives quite unreasonable and thus couldn't condone an act of self-destruction, much less assist its commission.

The second criterion isn't only about unreasonable motives. People can make bad choices for reasons that may initially look credible. For instance, it might make good sense for someone to choose to commit suicide on being diagnosed as having Lou Gehrig's disease, but it wouldn't make good sense for someone to choose to commit suicide because of the shock of being diagnosed as having diabetes. Diabetes is a disease that is treatable and usually allows people to lead fairly normal lives. It might look as if even a treatable disease suffices to warrant suicide if the individual in question greatly fears dependency, slow deterioration, and what they perceive as the stigma of chronic ill health. But a little reflection should show that something has gone seriously wrong if a person is ready to commit suicide when what they face is a situation that thousands of people find tolerable and which does not prevent them from enjoying full lives. People do lose perspective on their problems, and suicidal decisions or requests for assisted suicide may be prompted by unrealistic assessments of an illness's symptoms and consequences. If nothing else, the second criterion requires that there be consultation and time for reflection to enable a person to reach a rational decision.

The real problem posed by the second criterion's requirements regarding motivation isn't, as one might expect, the impenetrability of subjective feelings. Rather, it is determining if and when personal values and motives do properly outweigh common interests in survival and warrant suicide.[4] The importance of this determination is that suicide must be rationally motivated and warranted for assisted suicide to be permissible. Even if we relax our standards in recognition of the difficulty of truly knowing another's mind, as when we fail to really understand why someone wants to die, we must hold firm to the requirement that anyone assisting suicide has to agree that self-destruction is warranted. What is most unclear is how a potential suicidist's motivating values should be assessed when they run counter to what appear to be the person's best interests or are in line with those interests but misconceived. In this chapter we have to try to clarify the relation of personal motives to interests in the assessment of suicidal decisions and the permissibility of assisted suicide. We also need to consider if motives sometimes may be immaterial to decisions about assisted suicide. In the next chapter we look at interests.

ASSESSMENT OF MOTIVATING VALUES

From the perspective of the potential suicidist, the second criterion's job is to guard against self-destruction for inadequate or confused motives.

But from the perspective of others, the criterion is a crucial test of whether they may assist the commission of a self-destructive act. If the suicide that someone is asked to assist is motivated by values or priorities that the assisting person doesn't find cogent, providing assistance would be wrong.[5] The complication is that in medical contexts, an individual's motives may be overshadowed by prognostic factors.[6] This means that there may be good reasons, evident to others, why not continuing to live is in a patient's best interests. This amounts to the patient no longer having a real interest in survival that would be jeopardized by confused suicidal motives. It then looks as if, so long as the patient wants to die, personal motives are immaterial *whether or not they're cogent.* But it seems wrong to assist a suicide committed for significantly confused personal reasons, even if there are different, adequate reasons for suicide that are known to others. However practically efficient it may be, doing the right thing for the wrong reasons violates the principle of autonomy, because it isn't assisting someone's suicide for *their* reasons. In Kantian terms, it's to use a person as a means to an end.

The task of assessing a potential suicidist's motivation, in a medical context, is partly one of deciding how to give that motivation its due weight in situations in which external factors seem sufficient for the commission of suicide. The concern is that motivation may be seen as irrelevant to some decisions about assisted suicide because of hopeless conditions and prognoses. When that happens, there's a real danger that patients' requests for assisted suicide may be granted too readily. Admittedly, the purely practical difference here may be small, but too-ready accession to requests for assisted suicide may take us down the slippery slope to something much worse.

The basic test for determining whether one understands another individual's suicidal motivation, and whether that motivation is cogent, is to ask if one could reach the same conclusion in the same circumstances.[7] Anything less than this would seem to rule out assistance in suicide, since it is intuitively clear that people shouldn't help do something that they don't understand or consider wrong. However, this test takes us only a little way, because there is still a need for significant consensus among peers to satisfy the second criterion's requirements, and the test determines only individual assessments. The trouble starts when we try to forge a consensus from individual assessments. In trying to establish a consensus, we face two kinds of discrepancies: the expected disagreements about values, and the much more difficult disagreements having to do with value-priorities and how situations and agent-preferences are perceived.

The discrepancies occur because any two people either may not share the same values or may share the same values but disagree about their application. Discrepancies due to the holding of different values are beyond the limits of our project. The fundamental split here is between conceiving of life as an unrenounceable gift and conceiving of it as a possession falling under our discretion with respect to its preservation or abandonment. Our contribution to this debate is our criteria, which are offered to show that opting to die can be a rational choice and so should be tolerated by any rational value system. The discrepancies that concern us here are those having to do with the application of shared values.

Two or more parties to the consideration of assisted suicide may share values that permit self-destruction and agree that quality of life supersedes mere survival but disagree about whether in a particular case quality of life is bad enough to override the interest in survival and to warrant suicide. These discrepancies are also of two sorts: First, there are *normative* disagreements, in which a suicidist's peers judge that committing suicide in a given situation is understandable but immoral or irresponsible. The judgment might be: "Yes, given these motivating values and these circumstances, I might want to commit suicide, but I wouldn't because . . . ," after which would follow reference to moral obligations or prohibitions of suicide. The second sort of disagreement is one of perception. This is not normative but *cognitive* disagreement. Peers may judge that the importance the potential suicidist attaches to something is so out of proportion that it jeopardizes or precludes the rationality of suicide, and thus the permissibility of assisting suicide. Our interest is in this cognitive sort of disagreement.[8]

An example of cognitive disagreement is when someone asked to assist in suicide believes that a suicidist's concern about being a burden to their family during a protracted terminal illness is grossly exaggerated, given the family's economic situation and their willingness to care for the afflicted person. This is the kind of disagreement that may occur among people holding the same values, because the dispute is not about the values or even their relative ranking, but about whether a given value is being appropriately and reasonably applied. Here a peer's judgment might be: "Yes, given these values and these circumstances, I might choose to commit suicide, but . . . ," after which would follow a claim that the potential suicidist is, for instance, being morosely pessimistic and exaggerating the negative side of what they face.

Unfortunately, people seldom adequately consider the cognitive aspect of suicidal decisions, because they mistakenly see the question of whether to live or die as a pathological matter or as necessarily a moral one and therefore either dismiss the idea or assess suicidal deliberation purely in moral or normative terms. This means that peer assessment of suicidal motivation is often not a useful test but a foregone conclusion. However, the fundamental question the potential suicidist asks and must answer is not initially a moral one. The question is: "Do I prefer to live as I must, or to die?" As indicated earlier, it is only *after* that question is answered that other questions arise about whether one's moral code or obligations to others preclude suicide. It may well be that the answer to the question is: "I would prefer to die but can't because . . . ," but whatever moral considerations follow the "because" are secondary to the preference question. What makes things *look* different, and lends plausibility to the view that the decision is always a moral one, is that in our largely Christian culture, suicide is morally prohibited (for Catholics) or strongly disapproved of (by Protestants), either of which effectively precludes the preference question being asked. For most people in our culture, the question about their preference to live or die never arises, because prohibition or opprobrium regarding suicide makes their preference irrelevant.

Moral questions aside, what cognitive disagreements about suicide and assisted suicide come to is that even if values are shared, many see some lives as worth living that others see as unthinkable. The hard part is that these disparate judgments vary *within* the range of what is thought to be rational or reasonable in our culture or society, because what is at issue is not the underlying values themselves but their practical interpretation. A good example is how different people view dependency. Many put a high priority on being able to care for themselves, on not being dependent and a burden, and agree that unacceptable dependence may warrant suicide. But disagreement begins on what is or isn't unacceptable dependence. Few would disagree that dependence on some nursing care and regular treatment, e.g., insulin injections, doesn't warrant suicide, or that total immobility and complete dependence on a life-support system may well warrant suicide. But there would be a good deal of disagreement regarding any number of intermediate stages. For instance, those who agree that Lou Gehrig's disease warrants suicide at some point may not agree about when that point occurs. Some people might choose to die very soon after initial diagnosis; others might feel that doing so would be a pointless and possibly perverse waste of good time left.

CLINICIANS AND JURORS

Our second criterion addresses the extremely difficult question of when
a person's motivating values do warrant self-destruction, given the need
to respect and safeguard that person's interests. As we've indicated, it
also indirectly addresses the question of when motives may become
immaterial because of a patient's hopeless condition and prospects. Satisfaction of the criterion means that peers agree that in a particular situation, an individual's putting quality of life or another value ahead of
survival is a rational choice. And because the choice is rational in the
sense discussed earlier, the enactment of the choice merits assistance
when necessary. Peers also may conclude that at some point, so long as
an individual doesn't want to live under certain conditions, the situation
may make that person's motives immaterial to deciding whether to provide assistance in suicide.

Unfortunately, our standards for discerning flawed motivation are
considerably more elusive than those for discerning impairment of reasoning. The standards are largely transparent or tacit; they permeate
assessors' thinking rather than being readily articulable precepts. The
standards are internalized as people grow up in a culture, and then those
standards unreflectively determine what people consider reasonable and
what they reject as unreasonable.[9] This is how disagreement about motivation has to do with perception: The operant standards are not applied
in a reflective way; instead, they shape how a situation is perceived and
construed. Resolving this sort of disagreement between people isn't a
matter of articulating principles and arguing them out; it's a matter of
making a number of small and often unconscious adjustments in the
give-and-take of discussion and prompting similar adjustments by
others. Any consensus thus reached isn't unproblematic just because it's
a consensus, but neither is it merely an agreement reached by the few
people directly involved. That consensus has much more general force.
In reflecting the range of commonly held cultural and societal values
that determine what is and isn't reasonable, a particular consensus is
cultural and societal consensus writ small.

The parallel between this sort of consensus and juries working out
their verdicts is illuminating in two important ways. The first has to do
with what is commonly agreed on by members of a given societal and
cultural group; the second with views that characterize subgroups with

special interests. Appreciating both is crucial to understanding peer assessment of suicidal motivation in medical contexts.

In the case of juries, there are explicit standards in play: the law or laws that may have been violated and the judge's instructions. But jurors are counted on to apply tacit cultural and societal standards far broader than these standards, such as whether something was or wasn't a reasonable expectation on the part of a plaintiff or defendant. People selected to serve on a jury and asked to evaluate a problematic action as either in accord with or contrary to the law are selected to represent their society's norms in rendering a verdict. Aside from making judgments about society's explicit requirements and prohibitions, jury members apply their society's tacit norms by being products of that society. Part of the point of impaneling a jury is that its members are presumed not only to understand the applicable laws but also to embody our tacit norms. They are expected to apply those norms by construing and assessing situations as would the majority of society's members. Clinicians have special expertise regarding a potential suicidist's medical condition and prognosis, rather like jurors acquire some knowledge of the law. But also like jurors, clinicians embody and apply society's tacit norms.[10] And as with values, application of those norms may vary significantly, but without involving fundamental disagreement about the norms themselves.

Clinicians participating in appraisal of a request for assisted suicide function much like jurors: Individual assessments of something problematic are voiced and qualified in a dialogic process that results in a consensual decision. The theory is that the decision reached is not simply a result of mutual accommodation by particular participants but an achieved agreement with the representative weight of societal judgment. Supposedly, the rough edges of individual assessments, shaped by how shared values are interpreted and applied by each participant, are smoothed and made to fit with others to produce a common decision. The decision is common in both the sense that it is shared by the participants and in the sense that it represents what society at large would decide in the circumstances. Again like jurors, when clinicians decide to provide assistance in suicide, the decision is supposed to be one having the authority of communal judgment, not simply the weight of the opinions held by the individuals involved in the deliberation.

What complicates this idealized picture is the fact that there's more at work than shared norms or values. When juries are impaneled, prosecutors and defense attorneys work very hard to establish that jurors haven't already made up their minds about the case through special knowledge, bias, or inclinations prompted by their backgrounds or experience, since the whole point is that their judgments be impartial and based solely on evidence presented to them in court. Special knowledge can't be avoided when clinicians assess requests for assisted suicide, and it poses a difficult problem, since clinicians' assessments of requests for assisted suicide have to be considered unacceptably problematic if their knowledge significantly predisposes them to agree with the requests.[11] The trouble is that just as we don't want people serving on juries who've made up their minds about a case, we don't want clinicians participating in peer assessment of suicidal motivation if they're already convinced by a patient's chart that suicide is the patient's only sensible option. The danger is that such reliance on "objective" factors will cause insufficient attention to be paid to things such as confused motives.

It seems, then, that the most pressing issue with respect to application of the second criterion in medical contexts is that suicidal motivation may be too readily dismissed or discounted because of medical conditions taken to override motivational confusion on patients' parts. Assessment of the cogency of patients' reasons for suicide seems to be carried out not by their peers but by people whose experience, expertise, and special knowledge render them *un*representative of societal norms. As assessors, then, clinicians may very well make decisions that the rest of us wouldn't accept as representing our judgment about the rationality of suicide and the permissibility of assisted suicide.

THEORETICAL AND PRACTICAL PRIORITIES

As emerged in the last chapter, many of the elements in conflict between the requirements of ethical theory and the demands of clinical practice come together in the question of whether we should assess potential suicidists' specific lines of reasoning for choosing not to live or their general competence to make major decisions about their own treatment. This same question arises here, in connection with motivational assessment, so we need to say a bit more about the difference between assessing reasoning and general competence.

The contrast we've drawn so far is between focused assessment of the soundness of reasoning about self-destruction and broader assessment of the capacity to make responsible decisions about major treatment options. Assessment of reasoning is impersonal and noncontextual in the sense that it involves, first, determining that the reasoning isn't inconsistent, equivocal, question-begging, and so forth and, second, that it is free of factual error, false premises, and/or vitiating ignorance. The parallel is to assessing how someone does arithmetic. It doesn't matter, with respect to the correct answer, who happens to be adding a column of figures or in what circumstances they are doing the addition. Against this, assessment of general competence is always contextual, and the identity and particular circumstances of the person being assessed are central elements in the assessment. Another key difference is that while reasoning is assessed as either impaired or not, someone may be judged to be impaired in their reasoning some of the time but still competent to make major decisions about their treatment at other times. Someone's less than perfect reasoning may also be found acceptable when extenuating circumstances—e.g., great stress—are factored into the assessment. Standards for competence, unlike those for reasoning, aren't exact. Competence standards are patterns of judgment and behavior that society considers acceptable and reliable and that may be approached sufficiently closely, even if not fully met, for decisions to be found acceptably reasonable.[12] This is why when patients' general competence is assessed in medical contexts, the question asked isn't about specific formal and informal logical requirements but rather is: "Given their present condition and what they face, can we take them at their word about treatment options, or should we refer the matter to a surrogate decision maker?"[13]

Assessment of general competence is a more forgiving procedure than assessment of reasoning. The scope of what is considered relevant to assessment is much wider in the case of assessing competence, and individual elements in the assessment may be weighed against one another in ways that diminish the importance of the more problematic ones.

Serious impairment of reasoning is incompatible with general competence, so most clinicians believe that reasoning *is* adequately probed in clinical evaluation of the competence of patients requesting assisted suicide. Even though many theoreticians and some clinical ethicists don't think that suicidal reasoning is normally probed enough to satisfy the first criterion, it's undeniable that reasoning is probed to some degree in evaluating patient competence. However, motives are treated more circumspectly than reasoning in competence assessment, so the second criterion's requirements may be even less adequately met. First of all, we have a cultural tradition of taking motivating values and value judgments as unchallengeable,[14] much as we take taste preferences as unarguable. But more immediately relevant is that because patients' motivating values tend to be thought immaterial to treatment decisions to the extent that their medical conditions and prognoses warrant the treatment in question, patients' motives also may be thought immaterial to the assessment of requests for assisted suicide.

The thinking seems to be that it is relatively unimportant precisely *why* a patient wants not to live, if all indications are that continuing to live would mean only great and unrelieved suffering. A possibly confused reason for suicide, then, might be either ignored or thought no worse a motive, in the circumstances, than a hard-headed wish to avoid pointless agony. Impaired deliberation may be discounted to the degree that its suicidal conclusion is coincidentally what is thought to be in a patient's best interests. Provision of assisted suicide may be seen as justified by patients' prognoses and patients' actual desire not to live, as opposed to the motives that generate that desire. Clinicians may actually think it inhumane, or at least unnecessarily intrusive, to analyze patients' motivation when patients have every reason to want to escape tormenting situations.

Clinicians have a strong rejoinder to theoreticians' demands for strict interpretation of the second criterion and close analysis of suicidal motivation. The rejoinder is to ask about proposed alternatives to acceptance of patients' motives. If it is in a patient's best interests to be assisted in the commission of suicide, but the patient's motives don't satisfy the criterion, is it then a matter of helping the patient fashion better motives? Should attending clinicians inform patients that, at least as expressed, their motives fall short of acceptability, and then work with patients to formulate more satisfactory motives? What would be the point of such an exercise? Wouldn't it be merely to make everyone *else* feel better that patients committed suicide for reasons more acceptable to the rest of us? The only other alternative would be to deny patients' requests and possibly force them to endure long and agonizing deaths.

Clinicians' contact with patients who ask for help to die is contact with people in hopeless situations. Clinicians therefore find it difficult to think that if those people choose not to live, they should be prevented from taking their lives because their motives appear confused or implausible. Most clinicians working with the terminally ill are familiar with the rationalizations people produce to justify suicides that would have been unthinkable for many of them a short time earlier. What could be gained by destroying those rationalizations, if they don't indicate preclusive conditions such as clinical depression, and it's in the patient's interests not to live to endure greater suffering? It must be kept firmly in mind that for clinicians, the fundamental justification for a hastened death isn't found in their patients' thoughts or remarks; it's found in their patients' moribund and painfully deteriorating bodies.[15]

We might conclude that the motivation that the second criterion tests really doesn't matter in most clinical settings and that what does matter is to help patients die who don't want to live and who, because of their condition and prognosis, are better off not living.[16] If a patient's condition and prognosis warrant a hastened death, the patient's own particular reasons for wanting to relinquish life need be sufficient only *for the patient*. In short, peer assessment of motivation may be largely immaterial to the rationality of suicide in medical contexts. If so, the patient's own motives will be irrelevant to the permissibility of providing assistance in suicide, so long as it's clear that the patient chooses not to live.

However, the conclusion is disputable; it can be seen as tending to diminish patient autonomy. Recall that the relevant sense of *autonomy* is that of a free, knowing, and resolute choice or decision *in accordance with reason*. Autonomy may be seriously qualified if the decision to commit suicide is made for confused motives. Moreover, if we begin to waive patients' confused motives for what are thought to be good suicidal choices on other grounds, we risk paternalistically justifying actions for them that are ill conceived from their own perspectives.[17] Against this, it may be inevitable that compassion regularly forces indifference to confused motives and that such indifference is, in some cases, actually in keeping with the principles of nonmaleficence and beneficence[18] to a degree that overrides concerns about autonomy. It's just at this point that some see empathy playing its most crucial role, because empathic understanding of patients' situations, wishes, and needs could make the difference between paternalistically imposing a decision and making good sense of motivation that, though confused, actually serves a patient's best interests.

In the view of many, reference to empathic understanding adds little to claims that assisted suicide is warranted by patients' conditions, prognoses, and desire to die. Such reference is taken to mean only that attending clinicians feel compassion toward their patients. For the most part, compassion is considered a good but essentially extraneous—and possibly troublesome—emotion. To many, empathic understanding isn't perceived as any kind of relevant knowledge about others' motives or intentions because it isn't "scientific." Empathy is considered the intrusion of the passionate and impulsive into matters calling for cool, "objective" treatment. In medicine, there tends to be an excessive reliance on what can be quantified regarding a patient's condition and prospects, what can be annotated and tracked on a patient's chart.[19] With respect to assessing requests for assisted suicide, both clinicians and theoreticians are often inclined to think that it's actually wrong to adopt a potential suicidist's perspective to assess the rationality and advisability of self-destruction, because doing so violates the supposed objectivity of expert assessment.

Empathic understanding is especially relevant to motivation, because it's holistic or "nonlinear" in a way that contrasts with the "linear" assessment of reasoning. But this is not to say that such understanding is only a compassionate feeling. *Empathy*, as we are using the term, has a technical sense, as we indicated in chapter 1. The appeal isn't only what the dictionary defines as the ability to experience the feelings of another as one's own, though certainly that is part of it. For some, empathic understanding in the assessment of the permissibility of assisted suicide isn't merely a sympathetic grasp of someone's reasons for choosing not to live. That understanding is claimed to be a solid basis for making judgments about whether someone's motives warrant self-destruction and thus warrant assistance when those motives can't be realized without help. The point is that as a basis for those judgments, empathic understanding may be as sound as any claimed objective knowledge of patients' conditions. Ideally, empathic understanding of an individual's suicidal motivation would enable determination of whether that motivation warrants suicide despite appearing or being confused. Empathic understanding could complement prognostic grounds for assisted suicide and enable a positive decision by opening up more interpretive latitude for the appraisal of motivation than is allowed by more analytic assessment.

Support for the view of empathic understanding as knowledge is available mainly in recent work by feminist writers. These writers have focused on our culture's near obsession with scientific objectivity and its consequent negative attitude toward supposedly too subjective emotional elements in perception. Some of this work addresses the specific question of empathy's role in medical practice.[20] In medicine, as in other disciplines, practitioners see themselves as scientific and find it necessary to distance their professional judgments and practices from their emotions. Feminists denounce this aspiration to objectivity as misconceived and argue that in traditionally female activities, the dichotomy that produces the supposedly exclusive categories of the scientifically objective and the emotionally subjective isn't imposed to the same degree as elsewhere. But feminists also point out that this greater tolerance of "the emotional" in "woman's work" is due to that work being less valued than "objective" scientific work, "where *empathetic* knowing finds no place."[21] Feminist theorists argue that emotional experience yields real knowledge and affords reliable bases for action. They also argue that empathy serves to enhance understanding of complex matters.

Application of these arguments to the issue of assisted suicide is intended to show that empathy may help us to better understand suicidal motivation. When there is good, "objective" warrant for self-destruction to avoid great and unrelieved suffering, i.e., solid diagnostic and prognostic evidence, and the desire to die but for what appear to be the wrong reasons, empathy may demonstrate the adequacy of those apparently misguided reasons. For example, a patient may want to die to rejoin a long-dead spouse, convinced of the existence of an afterlife and seemingly ignoring the medical reasons for suicide. This is a motive for suicide that most theoreticians would find unacceptable. By obscuring or denying the possibility of death being personal annihilation, it blunts adequate awareness of suicide's consequences, thereby qualifying the rationality of the choice. Clinicians and some clinical ethicists would find the motive acceptable enough, arguing that empathic understanding could show it to be less a motive for self-destruction than an expression of the individual's having come to terms with impending death and wishing not to prolong the process.

The main problem posed by this view of empathic understanding has to do with confirmation. Whatever its faults, the scientific perspective's strength, and the force of its claim of objectivity, is that scientific knowledge stands or falls on repeatability and universality. That is, whatever is claimed to be scientific knowledge must be something that anyone can learn and apply successfully in similar circumstances. But claimed empathic understanding seems to allow too much latitude for cognitive disagreement regarding the interpretation and application of values. In other words, empathic assessments of motivation may result in disagreements that fall within the limits of what we consider reasonable regarding the application of shared values but still be contrary enough to block consensus in assessment. So judgment calls would still be necessary to resolve disputes about the adequacy of suicidal motives.

In the cases that concern us, those judgment calls would be made by clinicians. But it's possible for one clinician to claim empathic knowledge that a patient genuinely and rightly wants not to live, regardless of how inadequate the motives, and for another clinician to claim empathic knowledge that the inadequacy of the motives indicates deep and preclusive ambivalence. Empathic judgment seems to leave us with the original problem: the need to decide whether or not we can discount suicidal motivation at some point on the strength of diagnostic and prognostic considerations.

Empathic understanding can't be ruled out as a form of knowledge, and it's plausibly argued that it is just that, rather than being only emotional *rapport*. But questions do arise, particularly about why significant disagreements occur if empathic understanding *is* knowledge and how those disagreements are to be resolved.[22] The most worrying aspect of the resolution question is that with respect to the assessment of motives for suicide in medical contexts, and thus of the permissibility of lending assistance in suicide, it falls almost entirely to clinicians to resolve the disagreements. It is clinicians who conduct the assessments, it is clinicians who must decide whether or not to assist suicide, and it is clinicians who have the expertise to establish whether patients' medical conditions warrant suicide. This raises the issue of whether clinicians might not, as a group, be too inclined to dismiss problematic suicidal motivation because of their training and experience.

A TWO-EDGED SWORD

What is most central in this chapter are considerations that don't so much anticipate as initiate our discussion of the slippery slope argument. Whether or not we stress the more technical sense of empathy, assessment of general competence is largely empathic, because it's a function of the perceptions, sensitivity, and interpretive tendencies of those doing the assessing. Clinicians' decisions about patients' motives undeniably are made against a complex backdrop of professional and institutional norms, individual experience and expertise, and personal values and priorities. The question is whether we can count on those decisions being in line with broad societal norms and values and not representing only the special norms and values of the profession and individual clinicians.

Consider the likeliest way in which clinicians' decisions about assisted suicide may differ importantly from societal norms and values: Clinicians have ongoing contact with patients and observe their suffering; additionally, because of their experience and expertise, they understand their patients' prospects better than most of those patients do themselves. As a consequence, clinicians may make their assessments of patients' suicidal motives in ways that are too accommodating of patients' *expressed* desires to commit suicide. That is, they may not probe enough to determine that those expressed desires aren't motivated by something quite different from a desire to die, e.g., a need for reassurance even when little or none can be provided. Too-ready acceptance of expressed desires, and attendant acceptance of motives, may be the result of the mutually enhancing roles of human compassion and clinicians' expert knowledge of what patients face.

In assessing patients' suicidal reasoning, clinicians' personal value-shaped perceptions are clearly important, but they are much more important in assessing motives, because understanding another's motivation is by its nature a considerably more empathic exercise than understanding another's reasoning. The catch is that empathic understanding of another's situation is strongly conditioned by one's own priorities. As noted, the basic test for the cogency of suicidal motivation is whether one would make the same choice *oneself* in the same circumstances. However, given clinicians' experience and expertise, it's quite natural that they would incline more to committing suicide in circumstances similar to those of their patients than would the average member of our society. So, although experience and expertise enable more informed and objective assessment of requests for assisted suicide, they may tend to predetermine accession to those requests precisely because of better understanding of what is involved. The upshot is that fundamentally confused or misguided patients' motives may be taken as acceptable because they are perceived from a more informed perspective in which suicide is the most indicated option.

It will appear to many that most of the time clinicians will be right because suicide *is* the right choice. Nonetheless, we have to remember what was emphasized earlier: The fact that suicide is the rational choice in a given situation doesn't and shouldn't *compel* anyone to commit suicide. Autonomy requires that suicide be the individual's free choice, whether or not it is the most sensible choice. Even in a case in which suicide is clearly a patient's wisest course of action, and that patient expresses a desire to commit suicide, it is *still* necessary to assess the cogency of the patient's motives. If the motives *aren't* cogent, assisted suicide is not permissible, though voluntary euthanasia may be in order.[23]

The problem, then, is how we are to assess the acceptability of judgments made on bases that seem so vulnerable to professional inclinations. The parallel is to verdicts by jurors who know too much about one side of a case being tried. The very fact that clinicians differ significantly in knowledge and inclination from the rest of a societal population strongly suggests that peer assessment of suicidal motives at least can't be limited to attending clinicians. But the other side is that clinicians' knowledge and inclinations are the most relevant to the assessments that need to be made. What seems to emerge is that there's a fundamental split here. From a theoretical perspective, peer assessment of suicidal motivation must be based on broad cultural and social values. But the clinical reality is that assessment of suicidal motivation is based on expert knowledge of patients' conditions and prospects and on professional norms.

The point poses something of a paradox: We want clinicians to take the perspective of the detached observer in order to effectively apply relevant principles and expertise in making decisions about requests for assisted suicide. We also want clinicians to take the perspective of the empathically involved participant to better appreciate patients' needs and motives. This seems to be too much to ask, but we ask still more. We want training, expert knowledge, and clinical experience to inform clinicians' assessments and decisions. At the same time, we don't want training, expert knowledge, or clinical experience to skew clinicians' perceptions.

The problems faced in this chapter are several and appear intractable. First, it seems that patients' suicidal motives may not get even the relatively cursory attention that suicidal reasoning receives. Prognostic considerations may be taken as sufficient grounds for decisions about providing assisted suicide,[24] and patients' motives for wanting to die may be thought immaterial. The opposing point is the difficulty of putting aside pressing and sometimes overwhelming medical considerations for the sake of difficult detailed assessment of motives. Second, if empathic understanding is given a decisive role in decisions about assisted suicide, in order to mitigate both reliance on prognostic considerations and apparent motivational confusion, it's unclear what correctness criteria guard against clinicians' own interpretations of patients' situations skewing their decisions. The opposing point here is the risk of hamstringing clinicians with unworkable demands and regulations. Third, if strict application of the second criterion is required, to counter both overreliance on prognoses and possible overlooking of motivational confusion, we not only invite gross inefficiency but also may gain little or nothing, since deep probing of motivation will likely prove inconclusive too much of the time. The opposing point is that if we *don't* require strict application, we may open too wide a gap between expert assessment by clinicians and the peer assessment we've relied on to define rational suicide. That is, we may end up with a contextually determined sense of rational suicide that is possibly quite at odds with the wider societal sense.

As emerged in the last chapter, there are considerations for and against giving priority to theoretical requirements or to practical demands regarding the first criterion. It's arguable that the primary focus of assessment should be the potential suicidist's particular chain of reasoning. But it's also arguable that the primary focus should be the potential suicidist's general competence, because of practical obstacles to close analysis of reasoning and the likelihood that it will prove inconclusive too much of the time. With respect to the second criterion and the potential suicidist's motives, the focus issue resurfaces. However, although it's arguable that patients' motives for choosing suicide should be thoroughly analyzed, it seems more intuitively clear that if an individual is judged competent to make decisions about cessation of treatment or more intrusive actions,[25] and there are good medical reasons for cessation of treatment or those actions, then that individual's personal motives should simply be accepted. It seems reasonable to assume that if there is no cause to suspect underlying pathology, such as clinical depression, then acceptance of a patient as competent includes acceptance of the motivation they find compelling. For one thing, as noted earlier, it's sometimes hard to tell whether something is a *motive* for suicide or a rationalization of acceptance of impending death. Given good medical reasons for suicide, it would be counter to patients' interests to subject their personal motives to undue scrutiny.

One point worthy of reiteration has to do with a possible misimpression regarding assessment of patients' general competence. As we noted earlier, patients are assessed as competent or otherwise with respect to specific matters, such as providing informed consent for particular surgical procedures. And as we also noted, the judgment that a patient can choose responsibly to undergo or forgo a procedure is context-dependent, since a patient may be judged able to do so at one time but not another,[26] or with respect to one sort of decision but not another. The same is true regarding requests for assisted suicide. But despite this contextual specificity, assessment of competence is holistic precisely because the clinical evaluation deals with how and when the patient may be competent to make a responsible decision. This is how clinicians' assessment of patients' reasoning and motives contrasts most sharply with theoreticians' more or less context-free assessment of specific lines of reasoning or particular motives. What is assessed in medical situations is, first of all, a patient's capacity for making responsible decisions; only then is the question raised about the specific treatment decision. One of the things emerging here is that, given this approach, it may be that whereas confused reasoning is properly seen as a strong indication of likely incompetence,[27] confused motives perhaps should be less worrying. This is mainly because while we can't accept that *reasoning* is sound or not for particular individuals, we may need to accept that *motives* are adequate or not for particular individuals. We seem to be stuck with allowing the right action even if for the wrong reasons.

A QUESTION OF CATEGORIZATION

As indicated, clinicians' expert knowledge and experience is a two-edged sword. On the one hand, the combination enables them to make informed decisions about patients' requests for assisted suicide; on the other, it may color their assessments and decisions in ways that jeopardize the rationality of patients' suicides. Perhaps the best way to put the point is that if it is peer assessment that determines the rationality of suicidal motivation, the problem is that clinicians' aren't really patients' peers because of their expertise and inurement to dying. Against this is the admitted fact that we are inclined, and it appears rightly so, to be more yielding about the adequacy of personal motives for self-destruction when there is abundant independent evidence that it is a wise choice. It may be that part of the difficulty here has to do with how the category of assisted suicide is used.

One view is that hastening willing patients' deaths is assisting suicide, because the basic condition for those deaths being suicides is the patients' choosing to die. In this view, the question of agency is secondary to that of intention, in the sense that once a patient has expressed a desire to relinquish life, how death is actually brought about is not considered to materially affect its suicidal nature. For instance, whether patients die by being taken off ventilators[28] by clinicians or by taking a fatal dosage of something provided by clinicians does not matter as far as characterizating their deaths as assisted suicide. The thinking is basically that the expressed desire not to live under certain conditions is what matters, not precisely how that desire is achieved. The contrary view is that the category of assisted suicide should be used only in those cases in which patients themselves perform some act that directly causes death. In this latter view, taking a provided fatal dosage would be suicide, but requesting and being taken off a ventilator wouldn't be, because the patient is not the primary agent. Requesting and being taken off a ventilator could satisfy Beauchamp's requirement that death result from conditions "arranged by the agent," but the patient would have to be incapable in a practical sense of performing the necessary act. However, this isn't the place to try to sort out difficult questions about degrees of primary agency. What poses the most pressing problem here are the consequences of systematic misdescription of provision of aid in dying.[29]

Patients may express a desire not to live, on being given a forbidding prognosis. What they say may be merely an indirect request for reassurance or an ineffectual wish that things were otherwise, or it may be a genuine desire to die. But even if the latter, patients' motives may be problematic. For example, they may choose suicide less because of their impending future than because they feel that they *should* commit suicide in order not to be a burden, or they may see their prognoses as retribution for past wrongs and as a sign that they should sacrifice the time left them to atone for those wrongs and redeem themselves. Clinicians and clinical ethicists, who see the provision of requested aid in dying as assistance in commission of suicide, consider the responsibility for death in such cases to rest on the patients helped to die. Therefore, those patients' motives will likely be assessed fairly leniently. That is, since the patients in question are taken to be committing *suicide*, their motives are their business, so long as the patients are deemed competent. Motives, then, aren't seen as decisive with respect to whether or not assistance is provided. Against this, if clinicians see themselves as performing voluntary euthanasia, and thus bearing responsibility for causing death, they will want to assure themselves that the patients in question want to die for good reasons.

Given the nature of autonomy, some problematic motives could suffice to justify suicide and assisted suicide, but not voluntary euthanasia. For example, suppose a terminal patient having several months to live deeply resents and regrets being a burden to others at the end of life. The patient may decide to commit suicide rather than be a burden. We might have our doubts about this motive, but if the patient is competent, they have the right to end their life and even get help doing so. But if a patient asks for voluntary euthanasia in order not to be a burden, and clinicians accede to the request, that looks suspiciously self-serving. Though not a decisive point, most clinicians would think twice before causing the death of a patient for this particular motive, as opposed to assisting a patient's suicide for the same motive.

It may look as if we're splitting hairs, but the fact is that there are some things we can allow people to do, and even help people to do, so long as it is *they* who are doing those things. But if it is *we* who are asked to do those things, we might not be so willing to do them without better justification. The differences here are subtle, but they are important if what is at stake is someone's life. It is because of these elusive but significant differences

that theoreticians think that hastening willing patients' deaths is assisted
suicide only when suicide is rational according to strictly interpreted criteria. It's one thing to want not to live and to take one's own life, and quite
another to want not to live but to put the responsibility for causing death
on someone else. Wanting to relinquish life without the responsibility for
doing so is to desire euthanasia, not to intend suicide. If cases of what is
really voluntary euthanasia are regularly perceived and described as
assisted suicide, it is likely that responsibility for death will too often be
put on patients who neither want it nor can properly bear it.

One indication of the seriousness of the problem of categorization
can be found in how glossing the difference between assisted suicide and
voluntary euthanasia explains what initially looks somewhat odd. This is
how patients' reasoning and motivation can be subordinated to prognostic considerations without looking like violation of patients'
autonomy. Using the category of assisted suicide to cover cases of voluntary euthanasia appears to preserve patients' autonomy. Autonomy
actually appears to be enhanced when voluntary euthanasia is called
assisted suicide and is provided on the basis of prognoses and patient
requests or even merely their consent. Designating such cases "suicide"
makes the patient the primary responsible agent. In addition, it looks as
if patients' motives are fully respected because clinicians are unwilling
to challenge their free choices. But what worries theoreticians is exactly
that those choices may *not* be free, that they may be the products of confusion, undiscerned ambivalence, or contextual intimidation.

There's also a political advantage to generous use of the assisted-suicide category and avoidance of talk about even voluntary euthanasia.
Clinicians' traditional mandate has been to preserve life to the best of
their ability. Admittedly, they sometimes judge that it is best to allow (or
perhaps do more than allow) someone to die when treatment becomes
counterproductive, but since Hippocrates they have been constrained by
the nonmaleficence principle to at least do no harm. Yet now clinicians
are being asked to help their patients to die. This means that in many
cases they must bear the dual responsibility of deciding whether
someone is competent to choose to die and whether to help them do so.
Use of the category of assisted suicide in cases in which clinicians have
that dual responsibility emphasizes that it is *the patient* who is the primary agent, and that clinicians' participation is only one of facilitation,
thus deemphasizing clinicians' responsibility for patients' deaths.[30] However accurate or inaccurate this picture may actually be, it goes some
way toward easing the transition from clinicians as guardians of life to
sometime hasteners of death.

It may well be that in the majority of cases of requested assisted suicide in medical contexts, patients' motives for wanting to die are less important than they might be, not because prognostic or other factors are allowed to override those motives, but because they properly do so. In these cases, there is certainly contextual coercion in the form of human suffering, and it isn't clear that people in these punishing circumstances are even capable of adequate critical reflection on their own motives. Whether they say they want to rejoin a long-dead spouse or enter oblivion, they may just want to die and end their suffering. Nonetheless, it's important to determine if just wanting to die is preparedness to kill oneself, even if with help, or is the desire that someone else take one's life. If help in dying is requested, without specific suicidal intention, we're dealing with voluntary euthanasia. Motivation then calls for a different sort of evaluation, one considerably more dependent on diagnostic and prognostic factors. To gloss such cases as "assisted suicide" is to falsely attribute intent and capacity to patients who may be quite incapable of *self*-destruction.

Our consideration of the first criterion left us with many questions, but the most pressing is whether, in decisions about assisted suicide, we should assess patients' reasoning or patients' general competence. In looking at the second criterion and the matter of motivation, it seems that the required peer acceptance of patients' suicidal motives as cogent doesn't work very well in medical contexts. The critical factors appear to be the level of suffering and the nature of prognoses: The higher the suffering and the worse the prognoses, the less appropriate it seems to worry about what precise motives patients have for relinquishing lives that have become more than burdensome. We might conclude, then, that patients' desire to die is all that is needed when medical conditions indicate that death is in someone's best interests. The reservation is that we may have to be much more careful in our use of "assisted suicide" as a category for aid in dying. It may be that assisted suicide is a quite narrowly applicable category, one most correctly used when agents act primarily on their own and for sound motives. If so, voluntary euthanasia emerges as a more important category,[31] regardless of negative connotations and some clinicians' reluctance to accept more responsibility for causing patients' deaths. Motivating values have proved a difficult topic—one that raises hard questions about what goes on when patients are helped to die and how important personal motives are when weighed against minimal or nonexistent interests in survival. It seems that regardless of criterial requirements, when patients lose their interests in survival, a significant measure of discretion over the cogency of motivation is bestowed on those who assist at suicide or otherwise provide aid in dying in medical contexts. In the next chapter we look at the interests that are contravened by suicidal decisions.

SUMMARY

For suicide to be rational, a potential suicidist's motives for self-destruction must make good sense to others. There is need to guard against depression, morbid pessimism, or loss of perspective motivating someone to commit suicide when self-destruction is not warranted. But assessment of motivation is complicated greatly by both others' values and potential suicidists' circumstances. In the cases that concern us, clinicians' decisions about patients' requests for assisted suicide are colored by their own professional and personal priorities and by those patients' conditions and prognoses. These factors may unduly eclipse the motives being assessed, and those motives may then be too heavily discounted, too generously evaluated, or even ignored. Some think that empathic understanding by clinicians ensures that patients won't be either too hastily helped to die or forced to live longer than they want. But empathic understanding remains problematically subjective.

What seems undeniable is that suffering and hopeless prognoses increasingly render assessment of suicidal motivation pointless. We seem to end up with accession to requests for assisted suicide in medical contexts turning on prognostic considerations and the concurrence of patients. But some cases look dubious as instances of assisted suicide. The more reason there is to overlook the cogency of patients' motives, the likelier it is that the primary agency and responsibility for causing death have shifted to participating clinicians. This is because the reasons for not worrying too much about motives have to do with diminishing capacity for autonomous action on the part of patients, with patients' reluctance or inability to directly cause their own deaths, and/or with punishing circumstances that increasingly make motives immaterial. The question arises whether we're trying to make the category of assisted suicide do too much work. Though morally and politically more controversial, it may be that when patients' motivation becomes less and less material to clinicians' decisions about the provision of aid in dying, voluntary euthanasia is the more appropriate category.

NOTES

1. Note that our formulation doesn't speak only of motives but includes the values that underlie motives. To deal only with motives would leave untouched how a motive for suicide—for instance, wanting to avoid unnecessary suffering—arises from deeper values about the nature of human life.

2. This point immediately raises questions about subjective assessments of situations and personal autonomy. Some feet that it is simply impossible to adequately know another's mind, and that the judgment at issue can't be made with any authority and must ultimately be either paternalistic or arbitrary. This seems to us to be a naive view that exaggerates human subjectivity. We make judgments of this sort everyday when we think that someone is being foolish or obstinate. In most cases we can afford to let people do what they prefer and wash our hands of the matter, but this isn't the case with respect to self-destruction. Few reasonable adults would allow another human being to commit suicide for a reason they found absurd.

3. For instance, a patient, on being diagnosed as terminal, might respond with irrational anger at the unfairness of their situation That anger could be expressed as a decision to commit suicide to show everyone how little they care for a life suddenly limited by the diagnosis. Someone acting in this manner could be throwing away months or even years of worthwhile life.

4. See Prado 1990 for a detailed discussion of an extreme case—the Western perspective on the practice of *seppuku*.

5. The parallel is with someone being asked to assist in doing something they consider to be immoral or know to be illegal.

6. It goes without saying that prognoses change values and therefore a person's motives. However, the point here is the contrast and possible conflict between patients' value-dictated motives and clinicians' prognoses-dictated assessments. If a prognosis is bad enough, and a patient understands how bad it is, clearly the patient's assessment of the value of remaining life will come much closer to a clinician's more objective assessment. But the concern here is with the rather greater likelihood that this won't happen, and that the value a patient puts on remaining life will be considerably greater than the value put on that same life by a knowledgeable clinician.

7. Of course, "in the same circumstances" means sharing or empathically understanding the suicidist's values, since the point is to determine whether application of values held warrants self-destruction.

8. Recall that moral issues about suicide are secondary because they are contingent on application of particular moral codes.

9. As alluded to earlier, in our time we are very conscious of subjectivity, and are more ready to accept that something is or isn't thought reasonable by an individual.

10. Another important parallel between attending clinicians dealing with assisted suicide and juries is that in both cases the judgment delivered in effect recasts what was at issue in a newly determinate way. That judgment gives an act that was previously ambiguous a definite shape: In the case of a jury decision, after the verdict, something is or isn't a crime; in the case of assessment of suicide, after a determination on the basis of consensus, something is or isn't a warranted act of self-destruction.

11. Of course, in some cases that knowledge may prompt them to dismiss such requests out of hand. But what is more worrying is a too-ready accession to requests.

12. This is perhaps best illustrated by a judge ruling on the competence of an elderly person whose relatives feel that the person should no longer have control of finances. What the judge does is try to discern whether patterns of responsible behavior override the idiosyncratic or even inexplicable behavior that prompted the relatives' action, and the basic criterion is what most people would or wouldn't find acceptable.

13. To put the point in a rather cold-blooded, legalistic way, the question about general competence is at bottom a question of whether attending clinicians could be held negligent or otherwise at fault for accepting and acting on a patient's treatment-option decision. Age is a common deciding factor here. Physicians wouldn't accept a hospitalized nine-year-old's decision on whether or not to go ahead with some procedure, and in our culture, they'd tend to seek familial confirmation of a ninety-year-old's decision.

14. Most people would think that emergency-ward clinicians have neither the expertise nor the authority to dispute the religious or moral values behind, say, someone's refusal of a blood transfusion. They would think that instead of arguing with patients, which clinicians usually do, they should simply explain as carefully as possible the medical necessity of the transfusion.

15. Given the importance of Alzheimer's and other forms of dementia, "bodies" clearly includes "brains" here, though if the dementia were advanced enough, we would be dealing not with assisted suicide but with euthanasia.

16. As we consider later, this is where the question arises about the viability of the category of assisted suicide in medical contexts and where there is clear danger of assisted suicide sliding into euthanasia.

17. For instance, the medical condition and prognosis of a particular patient may be such that suicide is the wisest and most compassionate course of action. The patient may express the desire and intention not to live under the threatening circumstances. However, the patient's motives for choosing suicide may not be to avoid intense, unnecessary suffering. The patient may in fact prefer to endure that suffering for the sake of whatever time is left. But the patient may be convinced that clinicians and family *expect* commission of suicide to save everyone the financial and emotional costs of continuing to live. This is Caplan's fear about people expecting terminal and very elderly patients to do "the responsible thing" (Caplan interview on "The Kevorkian Verdict," *Frontline*, broadcast

May 14, 1996). In many circumstances, this would be a bad reason for committing suicide if it was an individual's main reason for doing so.

18. I.e., "do no harm" and "bring about good."

19. It's hardly only clinicians who are enamored of objectivity. The lure of the objective for theoreticians results in an inclination to rely too heavily on what can be propositionally stated. Contrary to this inclination is the relatively new and ongoing discussion in philosophy about the merits of narrative understanding of moral dilemmas and issues and of the inadequacy of purely propositional descriptions of such cases. See Prado 1984.

20. E.g., Nadelson 1993; Spiro et al. 1994; More and Milligan 1994; Code 1994.

21. Code 1994:72.

22. There is a parallel here to appeals to moral intuitionism. The question that arises regarding moral intuitionists' claims that we intuit what is right and wrong is why there are discrepancies. If the rightness or wrongness of an act is supposedly intuitively knowable, there should not continue to be disagreement. Such disagreement is most often attributed to factors that somehow occlude proper intuition, but that only pushes the problem back a step, since those who may be charged with occluded intuition can make precisely the same claim about their opponents.

23. In voluntary euthanasia, patients' motives play a less important part, because more of the responsibility for assessment of the rationality of the act is taken by participating clinicians. A request for *euthanasia*, as opposed to a request for assistance in the commission of suicide, is partial abrogation of responsibility by the patient.

24. One irony is that, in some cases, taking prognostic considerations as decisive and largely ignoring patients' motivation may be a result of greater rather than lesser empathic involvement with patients. That is, clinicians may be blinded by what they perceive as a patient's agonizing condition and want to end the pain at all costs, perhaps seriously underestimating the patient's willingness to bear that pain to continue to live.

25. That is, as opposed to a close family member or possibly a government board or appointed individual bearing the responsibility of making the decisions and signing the requisite forms.

26. For instance, a certain period of time may need to be allowed after the administration of medication.

27. Consider that it might be decided that although an individual is not generally competent but is able to reason clearly in certain circumstances, suicide may be warranted, and the persons's lack of competence may itself be a reason supporting suicide.

28. We use the more current term *ventilator* instead of *respirator*.

29. There's also a problem about autonomy, specifically, the measure of the autonomy of which patients are capable. Terminal, very elderly, and severely disabled patients may simply not be capable of fully autonomous decisions, *even*

though they are judged competent to make treatment decisions in the eyes of the law and most medical institutions. The incapacity is due to a combination of things: stress, debility, the effects of strong sedation, the confusion attendant on being hospitalized, and so on. According to law and institutional policies, if patients are judged competent, clinicians are bound by those patients' decisions. But the reality may fall well short of the legal fiction.

30. This is why opponents of legalized assisted suicide attempt to gloss the difference between assisted suicide and euthanasia. They want to focus on the authority that legalization would confer on clinicians to take life, as opposed to only assisting its abandonment.

31. Part of our point in providing bibliographic material on media coverage of aid in dying is to demonstrate how "assisted suicide" is the description of choice in discussing both policy and particular cases regarding aid in dying. Couching the public debate in terms of assisted suicide, as opposed to voluntary euthanasia, is decidedly less alarming, because assisted suicide doesn't invite or suggest what opponents like to play on: the idea that once *voluntary* euthanasia is sanctioned, *involuntary* euthanasia will soon follow.

5

THE INTEREST IN SURVIVAL

The third criterion is designed to prevent personal values from overriding an individual's best interests. The criterion requires that "suicide [be] in the agent's interests, not causing more harm than continuing to live." The typical situation the criterion guards against is someone choosing to die because they value something, e.g., quality of life or personal honor, more than their continued survival, but where that valuation is excessive relative to their interest in continuing to live. In this way, the third criterion complements the second, differing only in focus. The second criterion protects the importance of personal values against assumptions about the interest in survival; in particular, against the widespread view that personal values and priorities are automatically overridden by either the interest in survival or its lack.[1] The third criterion protects interest in survival against problematic personal and communal values and priorities. With respect to assisted suicide in medical contexts, the third criterion also protects against interest-eroding influences on suicidal deliberations and choices. This extended protection is necessitated by the combination of patients' vulnerability and clinicians' authority. It's not our intention to suggest that clinicians pressure their terminal, very elderly, or severely disabled patients into suicide, but as we saw in the last chapter, patients' confused suicidal motives may be discounted for no worse reasons than compassion for those whose suffering appears to outweigh the worth of the short time left to them. In a similar way, inadvertent or unconscious influencing of patients' decisions may occur because of compassion or, as we'll see below, how clinicians perceive patients' situations. Whatever the reasons, and regardless of how unintentional it may be, influencing of patients can be very powerful. After all, a *physician* suggesting to—or merely agreeing with—a patient that suicide may be a wise choice "is very coercive."[2]

The issue in the last chapter was about patients wanting to commit suicide or requesting assisted suicide for confused motives, and whether their confused motives should or shouldn't count against provision of assisted suicide. That issue is essentially about the acceptability of clinicians helping patients do the right thing even though patients are doing it for the wrong reasons. In this chapter we face something different, namely, the extent to which judgments that patients' have little or no interest in survival should influence clinicians' decisions about providing assistance in suicide. A related question is the extent to which clinicians' judgments should influence patients' deliberations. The issue is essentially about how clinicians' convictions about what is the right thing to do in given cases relate to patients' decisions, and the extent to which those convictions determine what clinicians themselves do. This isn't a matter of clinicians dealing with patients in malicious or even merely insensitive ways; the concern is just the opposite, namely, that compassion might move them to act in ways contrary to patients' autonomy: "[t]he very idea that one might *fall victim* to well-intentioned care providers who could impose their judgments upon a service recipient now strikes us as frighteningly real."[3]

In the cases that concern us, the worry is not only that an interest in survival might be taken as overriding patients' wishes to relinquish life but also that negative assessments of patients' interests in survival may cause clinicians to unduly influence patients and/or detrimentally affect their treatment decisions. Undue influence would most likely be exerted by how prognostic considerations are presented to patients and how much they are told about life-prolonging but costly treatment options.[4] As for detrimental effects on treatment decisions, the likeliest problem is that decisions negatively affecting patients may be made and not adequately conveyed to them, despite legal and professional requirements that significant treatment decisions involve patients' consent.[5] In this chapter, then, we don't only examine the third criterion's interests requirement for rational suicide; we also move closer to discussion of the slippery slope issue.

Patients may immoderately discount their own interest in survival. That would be the main problem here, if we were dealing simply with suicide. But we're dealing with *assisted* suicide in medical contexts. The main problem, then, is how clinicians' assessments of patients' prospects may breach the third criterion's requirement that suicide not do more harm than good by contravening interests. The key point is that there are no decisive independent standards for assessing interest in survival. Regardless of patients' actual medical conditions and prognoses, how patients and clinicians *perceive* continued life in critical medical circumstances is central to assessing patients' interest in survival. Some terminal patients may unduly discount the worth of a few weeks or even days of life, just as others may put too high a value on living as long as possible because they are driven by such things as religious beliefs or simply wanting to be around for a specific event, such as the birth of a grandchild. For their part, clinicians have traditionally been committed to prolonging life as long as possible, so they may overestimate their patients' interest in survival. However, as is becoming increasingly likely, clinicians may discount too heavily the time left to patients. A few days, even a month or two, may look insignificant to attending clinicians with futures measured in decades. It may appear reasonable to them for patients to sacrifice that brief time for the sake of a more comfortable death and avoidance of further suffering, or perhaps to not further drain scarce resources. But from patients' perspectives, even a few days may appear precious and worth enduring even acute suffering. Though patients' survival time in the relevant cases may be quite short, it is all the time those patients have left. Therefore, suicide may be rendered irrational if patients are unduly influenced to discount their interest in survival, either by how their prospects are presented to them by attending clinicians or by treatment decisions incompletely or misleadingly communicated to them "for their own good."[6]

Hopeless prognoses and intense suffering can make it look as if only misplaced sentiment or foolishness could prompt anyone to think that a patient's suicide could contravene a significant interest in survival. Requests for assisted suicide, whether or not unduly influenced, may look too propitious to probe too deeply. However, a healthy clinician's perception of the value of a few days or weeks is likely to be very different from a patient's perception of that same time, and brevity of survival time sacrificed isn't sufficient to justify suicide or to legitimate assistance in commission of suicide. Despondency or bravado can make someone throw away life made all the more precious by its brevity. Too-ready accession to requests for assisted suicide may render assisted suicide wrong even if the life forfeited is measured in days or possibly hours. The trouble is that there comes a point when we change over from seeing someone as terminally ill to seeing that person as clinging to life. As often as not, there's a measure of disapprobation involved in the change. It's as if we feel that at that point any reasonable person would value dignity and release from suffering more than the little time they may have left or that technology might grant them. In those circumstances, we are inclined to take requests for assisted suicide at face value. But this is something we need to resist because of what we may be doing to ourselves. It's just at those times when someone seems to have no appreciable interest in survival that we have to pause and consider if we're missing something, if only because we can't allow ourselves to slip into helping others to die just because they ask us to and *we* think they should. Suicide still has to make sense for anyone to assist its commission, and slippery slopes are paved with well-intentioned assumptions that because *we* think someone should relinquish life, *they* must want to relinquish life.

What makes all the difference, in the sense of resolving possible doubts, is the degree of suffering.[7] If an individual's pain is great enough and irremediable, then the chances of wrongly acceding to a request for assisted suicide seem to reduce to near zero. Clearly, the chances of contravening someone's interest in survival decrease proportionately when survival offers only more pain.[8] The crux of the matter can be put in terms of actual and expected suffering superseding agent-based rationality requirements. That is, when suffering is great enough, adherence to the criteria for rational suicide could become inimical to someone's welfare if the criteria continue to be applied primarily from that someone's perspective. This is not to say that suicide no longer need be rational; it is to say that its rationality ceases to be determined from the suicidist's or patient's point of view. Suicide must still be in the patient's interests, it must still do less harm than continuing to live, but that determination is no longer made on the basis of the patient's own perception of their interest in survival. Just as patients' motives for dying may become immaterial in bad enough circumstances, patients' own perceived interests may become immaterial in the same circumstances. It may, in effect, cease to matter what patients think about what's best for them when their situations are desperate enough.[9]

This shifting of the interest assessment from patients to clinicians is ill advised in many cases, and it's a dangerous move of precisely the sort that adherents of the slippery slope argument fear. It's a move that, though sometimes justified, could easily be an abrogation of patients' autonomy and responsibility. But when the shift *is* justified, we're no longer dealing with assisted suicide but with voluntary euthanasia. In other words, if the suffering level is high enough to warrant ignoring patients' own perceptions of their interests, as well as their motives, in acceding to requests for assisted suicide, the suffering is also high enough to render problematic patients' capacity to commit rational suicide. Assisted *suicide* requires that patients' choices be autonomous and rational. If patients are suffering so much that clinicians can allow medical considerations to override any possibility that requests for assisted suicide conflict with patients' perceptions of their own interests,[10] then what clinicians are acceding to are simply requests for termination of life, which are requests for voluntary euthanasia, not assisted suicide. Quite aside from questions about perceived interests, the telling point here is that the patients in question aren't concerned with being primary agents and causing their own deaths; they just want their tortured lives to be over, regardless of who actually causes death.

The theory-practice conflict comes to something of a head here. Clinicians will argue that only someone unfamiliar with serious human suffering could insist on an assessment of how patients perceive their interest in survival when they are wretched enough to ask for assistance in suicide. The view is that patients' negative perceptions of their interest in survival are plainly evident in their demeanor and requests. The contention is that it's solicitude for patients that prompts accession to requests for assisted suicide, that great suffering and hopeless prognoses clearly warrant patients' sacrificing their short and blighted futures. Clinicians feel that the cases in question leave no room for quibbles about rational choices or whether a merciful death is assisted suicide or voluntary euthanasia. Clinicians believe that their experience proves that a few more days or weeks of life often aren't worth what must be endured to realize them.

In both prudential and moral terms, this is a utilitarian judgment. Its force is that the value of continued life may be outweighed by the conditions under which that life must be lived. Utilitarian judgments require crucial assumptions about consequences.[11] Although sound judgments can be made, no one can know with certainty that a patient's condition may not improve or be adapted to in ways that make it more bearable. This possibility increases in proportion to the amount of time a prognosis offers. The longer the projected survival time, the stronger the possibility that things could get better. In addition, regardless of how humane and well-intentioned, clinicians' judgments are third-person ones; they're judgments about what is best *for someone else*.[12] That's why patients' perceived interest in survival must be discerned and taken into account, regardless of what patients may say in moments of weakness or despondency. Clinicians also must be sensitive to deeper problems underlying even repeated and apparently heartfelt requests for aid in dying.[13] However, beyond their charts, test results, and professional assessments, attending clinicians can go only by what their patients say to them. And clinicians, being as human as their patients, may interpret a request for assistance in suicide as more resolute than it is, especially when the requesting patient's condition is such that the clinicians wouldn't want to live if in the patient's place. Clinicians may too readily assume that patients' understanding of the utilitarian equation is the same as their own. So we seem to have an intractable problem. It's hard to see what might give clinicians better access to patients' own perceived interest in survival; yet there's reason to believe that what patients say when they ask for assisted suicide might not be enough, and that what clinicians hear, through their compassion and expertise, might be too much.

What we need here is greater clarity on what might be underestimated, if not contravened, when clinicians accede to problematic requests for assisted suicide. We can begin by sorting out the cases in which such requests may be made. There are several possibilities generated by the intersection of two main kinds of cases: cases ranging from patients who are relatively free of serious suffering to those who are suffering considerably, and cases ranging from patients whose prognoses indicate very brief remaining life to those whose prognoses indicate fairly substantial periods of expected life. Intersection of these two general kinds of cases results in four more specific sorts of cases that provide important reference points: first, there are cases in which patients are suffering and have only days or even hours to live; second, there are cases in which patients are suffering and have considerable time left to live; third, there are cases where patients aren't suffering and have a very short time left to them; and fourth, there are cases in which patients aren't suffering and have weeks or months left to live.[14] Suicide and provision of assisted suicide are most readily justified in the first type of case.[15] In the second sort of case, suicide and assisted suicide may be nearly as easily justified if prognoses offer too little hope for improvement in the time available. In the third sort, suicide and assisted suicide make little sense from either the patient's or the clinician's perspective, and attempts to justify the latter would look like yielding to expediency. In the fourth case, it may be quite difficult to justify suicide or assisted suicide, because patients' interests in survival are greatest.

Though clearly more so in the third and fourth, there may be a conflict of patients' and clinicians' values in all four sorts of case. To some—both patients and clinicians alike—serious suffering together with little time left justifies suicide and assisted suicide, whereas reasonably bearable suffering[16] and fairly significant time left tend to preclude the advisability of suicide and assisted suicide. To others, such considerations as quality of life, independence, and the desire to be free of even bearable pain suffice to justify suicide and to permit assisted suicide even when suffering is tolerable and there's significant time left. The trouble starts when patients and attending clinicians differ on these views. One kind of conflict occurs when a patient who isn't suffering much and has a good deal of time left wants to commit suicide, but attending clinicians think that the patient is being foolish or inordinately pessimistic. Another kind occurs when a patient who's enduring terrible suffering and has very little time left refuses to consider any sort of hastening of death, and attending clinicians think that assisted suicide or voluntary euthanasia is the most indicated course of action.[17]

Patients who are enduring tolerable suffering and have weeks or months of life left to them but want to commit suicide are cases of "presurcease" suicide, because they fall into a murky area between surcease suicide and preemptive suicide.[18] In other words, they fall somewhere between death being an escape from immediate and unrelenting torment, and death being a way of avoiding threatening but not yet actual torment. These ambiguous cases most clearly show the diversity caused by patients' differing perceptions of their interests in survival. Two patients, both enduring tolerable pain and both having substantial time left to live, may differ radically regarding self-destruction. One may want to commit suicide because the time left looks worthless; the other may want to live because the time left looks precious. But in these cases, it is unlikely that attending clinicians will think that self-destruction is advisable. Precisely because the suffering being endured is tolerable, and there is significant time left, we would be suspicious that a clinician encouraging suicide was more concerned about the difficulty or cost of care than the interests of the patient.

Things get tricky when patients' perceived interests in survival either compound reasonably tolerable physical suffering with intolerable psychological suffering or make intolerable physical suffering somehow bearable. In short, clinicians' assessment of patients' circumstances as tolerable or intolerable may be qualified, if not invalidated, by patients' attitudes toward their own suffering and prospects. For instance, a patient in great pain and with very little time left may be determined to live every moment possible.[19] Here the patient's perceived interest in survival confounds clinicians' compassionate and expert judgments that, given the patient's circumstances, either assisted suicide or voluntary euthanasia is most indicated.[20] Another patient enduring fairly mild pain and having months to live may be equally determined to commit suicide.[21] Here the patient's perceived interest in survival also confounds expert judgments that, given the patient's circumstances, neither assisted suicide nor voluntary euthanasia is indicated. In the first case, clinicians may be inclined to influence the patient to consider suicide or voluntary euthanasia. This may be done quite subtly and even inadvertently. It is more likely that clinicians will readily fasten on a wish for death expressed while the patient is in a particularly despondent mood. Even if there's no request for assisted suicide by the patient, or only passing reference to it, clinicians may begin to project a wish for death onto the patient.

Once there are good medical reasons for the question of self-destruction to arise, perception of these cases by some attending clinicians may tend to be that the patients concerned no longer have an interest in survival significant enough to make it worth bearing present and projected suffering. If the patients disagree, clinicians will likely think that it is only because they either haven't grasped the seriousness of their prognoses or entertain vain hopes of miraculous improvement. Talk of an interest in survival, then, rings hollow to clinicians at the point when death intrudes as the most sensible alternative to agonized life. And it is just at this point that clinicians feel most distant from theoreticians' requirements concerning the rationality of suicide. Some suffering patients are seen as no longer having an interest in survival significant enough to require showing death to be a rational option, because it has become the only option.[22] Some clinicians feel that no one lacking ongoing contact with actual patients can understand how evident it can be when death is the only choice. However, it's precisely these cases that concern theoreticians regarding conflicts between clinicians' assessments and patients' autonomy. The reason is that, as we've just seen, patients' perceptions of their own interests in survival may differ markedly from clinicians' assessments and be discounted or ignored.

Unlike some adherents of the slippery slope argument, most theoreticians don't think that clinicians will kill resisting patients on the basis of their own convictions. The serious concern is about unduly influencing highly vulnerable patients or precluding some of their options by making treatment decisions that may be incompletely or misleadingly communicated to patients "for their own good." An additional concern for theoreticians is the effect of clinicians' familiarity with, and even inurement to, death and dying. The undeniable fact is that regardless of empathic understanding, there is an irreducible difference between patients' and clinicians' perceptions of patients' interests, and clearly both expertise and experience, or their lack, strongly color these respective perceptions. This means that mechanisms are necessary to ensure that an acceptable balance is maintained in the weight given both sets of perceptions in making treatment decisions and, as important, in formulating questions about treatment are formulated and putting them to patients. However, it's still unclear just what is at issue when these perceptions conflict. We've spoken of patients' "perceived interests," but now we need to delve deeper into what these are and what they contrast with when there are conflicts.

INTERESTS

What is weighed in suicidal deliberation is not the value of being alive against the value of being dead, since the latter is not a state at all and so cannot be evaluated.[23] Instead, what is weighed is an individual's willingness to endure certain conditions against death as the cost of *not* enduring those conditions. As Battin puts it, assessment of whether suicide is in or contrary to one's best interests is a matter of assessing what must be borne in continuing to live, and whether its being borne is made worthwhile by "important experience during the pain-free intervals."[24] The interest in survival is not an interest in bare survival for its own sake. To retain life is to remain capable of valued experience, so the utilitarian assessment, whether moral or prudential, is always one of what must be borne to preserve that capability, and whether what must be borne outweighs even the best experiences that can be anticipated.

Much of the point of the last chapter had to do with deciding when personal values warrant self-destruction. The main concern was to ensure that potential suicidists' motives for ending their lives made good sense, since the second criterion requires that a suicidist's values not unduly contravene that person's interests. The heart of the matter was that potential suicidists' peers should agree that suicidists' value-determined motives for dying warrant contravening their common interest in continued life. Balancing the second criterion, the third enables judgments that qualify the importance of potential suicidists' values to protect their interests. However, in medical contexts, the third criterion may appear redundant when someone's interest in survival has been reduced to near zero or turned negative, in that surviving is against the person's interests because it offers only suffering. In the last chapter we were left with the question of when patient motivation is sufficiently reduced in importance, by suffering and prognostic considerations, to be rendered immaterial to decisions about providing assisted suicide. Here it seems that patients' interests may be reduced in importance by the same factors. But in the cases that concern us, we have to deal with *two* different perspectives on the interest in survival, those of patients and those of clinicians.

Interests are of different sorts and of varying significance. We speak of something being in our interests in a number of importantly different senses, two of which are crucial to our discussion.[25] One sense of something being in our interests simply has to do with what we want. If we want something, it's in our interests to get it, since we have an interest in getting what we want. This sense of "in one's interests" is neutral with respect to whether what we want is good for us, or, alternatively, it sometimes implies that if we want something badly enough it takes priority over what's good for us. This first, or "want," sense of something being in one's interests needs to be acknowledged, because it's perhaps the most commonly used sense, but it isn't relevant here. The reason is that this sense mainly has to do with wanting something in an unreflective way. It's possible that someone might want to die in this sense, but we are dealing with choosing to commit suicide, and to be rational, doing so must be reflective.

A second sense of "in one's interests" is one that certainly concerns us and contrasts with the "want" sense. It has to do with something being in one's interests from one's personal-value-laden perspective. Something that is in one's interests in this sense isn't something that is simply wanted; it is something wanted because one's values determine its priority in the hierarchy of desires that in part define an individual's personhood. This sense is central to disputes about suicide, because as we saw in chapter 4, interests determined by value-laden perspectives may oppose and in some cases override the interest in survival. For instance, it may be that suicide is in someone's interests in this value sense if, from their perspective, it is better to die an honorable death than to live in shame. This value sense contrasts with the want sense of "in one's interests," because what is in a person's interests in this sense need not be what the person actually desires. Someone who firmly believes that it is better for them to die an honorable death than live in shame may not actually want to die but may choose to die to satisfy the demands of their person-defining values. We'll call this the "value" sense of "in one's interests."

A third sense of something's being in one's interests is also highly relevant here, and it is when something is judged to be good for us but either is not wanted or is not wanted enough, though it is acknowledged as possibly or even clearly desirable. For instance, smokers may recognize that it's in their interests to stop smoking, but they simply may not want to stop or may prefer the pleasure of smoking to the abstract possibility of better health and longer life. This sense of "in one's interests" is referred to in what follows as the "prudential" sense, and as we'll see in a moment, it is often at odds with individual priorities. The reason why is that the prudential sense is the communal version of the individual value sense. The value sense captures what is in the interests of a given individual as determined by that person's values. The prudential sense captures what is judged to be in *anyone's* interests as determined by a community's values, culture, and history. *Community* here may refer to the whole of humankind, as when the interest in survival is judged to be a universal human interest. This is how prudential interests come to be considered objective interests that are independent of personal values.[26] This is also the basis for the strongest claim made against the second criterion, which is that motivating values can never override the interest in survival, because suicide is never in one's interests in this supposed objective sense. This argument holds that suicide at most may appear to be in one's interests in the want sense or value sense, but that neither of these suffices to warrant self-destruction.

When we speak of prudential interests, in this chapter and later, and contrast them with value interests, we don't mean to suggest that prudential interests are objective or universal. What we mean by prudential interests is whatever is determined to be in someone's interests on the basis of the broadest communal consensus. Reference to *prudential* interests is also an indirect reference to those interests that are in fact most people's *value* interests, that is, what most people perceive as their interests.

Recourse to prudential interests in the present context is the attribution to human beings of a common interest in continuing to live, but that interest doesn't have to be something mysteriously independent of our values, such as life being an unrenounceable gift of God. Prudential interest in survival need be based only on the understanding that since life is the precondition of all value, and life is irrecoverable once lost, it suffices that a person *is alive* for that person to have an interest in continuing to live. To be able to attain value is itself desirable and needs no justification. What needs justification is forfeiting the ability to attain value. Human life, then, doesn't require justification for its continuance; what is required is justification for its willful abandonment. To appeal to a prudential interest in survival, when debating the rationality of someone's suicide, is minimally to question the adequacy of that person's reasons for self-destruction from a communal perspective. We can proceed on the basis that to maintain that there's a prudential interest in survival is to put the onus for justifying suicide on those who would forfeit their lives. With this stipulation, we avoid bogging down in inconclusive discussions about whether or not there are objective or ahistorical interests. The prudential interest in survival can be taken as basically requiring that we be able to say how an individual is better off relinquishing life than continuing to live, because that individual requires no special reason to stay alive. We can also proceed on the basis that to refer to value interests, particularly value interests in continued life, is to take up individuals' personal perspectives on their own survival. As has clearly emerged, value interests and prudential interests may differ significantly in any given case.

INTERESTS AND PERCEPTIONS

Having clarified the senses of "in one's interests" that concern us, the next step is to see how the prudential interest in survival may be jeopardized or contravened in cases of assisted suicide in medical contexts.

One threat to rational suicide posed by value interests, as described in the last section, is that individuals may fixate on certain features of their situation and not give due weight to a still significant interest in continued life. Put in terms of prudential interests, the danger is that inadequate reasons for self-destruction will be taken as overriding prudential interests because of some judgment-skewing factor, such as an overly pessimistic view of a medical prognosis or possibly of how one will deal with what the prognosis threatens. Perhaps the most common sort of case is one in which people receiving terminal prognoses are so overwhelmed by the prospect of death that they too readily discount the value of any life left to them. Individuals' perception and assessment of the future may be as much distorted by the shock of their prognoses as by a condition such as clinical depression. Patients told that they have only months or even a year or two to live may hastily dismiss the worthwhile experiences those months or years may hold and decide that they'd rather die immediately than be haunted by knowledge of impending death. Patients may also misperceive their own past values and preferences. Previously highly prized contact with family, or gratification gained from creative work, may suddenly seem of only marginal value and be dismissed as not worth living for.

To ensure that potential suicidists fully appreciate their prudential interest in the time they may hastily decide to forfeit, what has to be argued is not an abstract claim about life's sanctity but that it's worthwhile to continue to be able to attain value. As we noted earlier, it is unproblematic that value is desirable; it clearly follows that it is desirable to be in a condition to attain value. However, as we've seen, the complication in medical cases is that we must deal with more than potential suicidists' own assessments of the future. In medical contexts, clinicians are also involved in the assessment, and they may believe strongly that patients' futures are such that whatever value may be attained will be outweighed by suffering. That's why an attending clinician may accept a patient's request for assisted suicide without enough probing. If a clinician firmly believes that even an ambivalent or inadequately reflective suicidal decision is in fact the wisest choice, why probe the reasons for the request and possibly introduce not only more ambivalence but also greater delay? But what can go wrong in these cases is that the various factors that condition and jointly determine clinicians' judgments may be slanted against the patients' value interests, and possibly even their minimal prudential interests, by the special character of clinicians' training and experience, as well as the institutional policies and priorities with which they work.

The majority of suicides in medical contexts are surcease suicide: suicide opted for and committed in the face of present suffering, as opposed to feared or anticipated suffering, and in light of a hopeless future, as opposed to one offering some chance of betterment.[27] The consequence is that, as we noted before, application of the criteria for rational suicide is bound to be seen as declining in importance as patients' conditions and prospects worsen. As emerged in the last chapter, potential suicidists' motives may become essentially immaterial and their rationality, in effect, irrelevant, given high enough levels of suffering and hopeless prognoses. The rationality of suicide as an option may seem to become more evident and compelling, and more removed from patients' own reasoning and deliberation, as suffering increases and hope for improvement decreases. What this amounts to is that suicide appears to become more rational as an option as prudential interests diminish. However, *value* interests may not decrease in line with prudential ones, and this sets the stage for conflict.

The question that emerged in the last chapter is how we can tell, in cases in which patients' level of suffering is less than decisive, when patients' suicidal motives cease to matter to clinicians' decisions about assisted suicide. Retrospectively, we can reformulate the question as being about when the reduction of prudential interests renders the motives behind requests for assisted suicide immaterial to decisions about its provision. The question in this chapter has to do with how value interests are affected when prudential interests become minimal or turn negative.

However, things are getting complicated, and we need to keep clear about the roles of reasoning, motives, value interests, and prudential interests. Before continuing with difficult matters that may be easily misconstrued, we should recap just a bit.

As we saw, application of the first and second criteria involves assessment of impairment and evaluation of the importance of individuals motives with respect to clinicians deciding to provide requested assistance in suicide. But in both cases, we took it that patients request that assistance. The issues had to do with whether those requests were based on proper reasoning and cogent motives. It bears reiterating that, with respect to the motives considered in the last chapter, the issue wasn't about patients *not* wanting to commit suicide but about their wanting to commit suicide for the wrong reasons. The question then was whether confused reasons should count against clinicians deciding to provide assistance in suicide. The present issue is in some ways similar but is still importantly different; it is basically about clinicians' negative assessment of patients' prudential interests in survival *influencing* patients' decisions and requests and thereby possibly contravening patients' value interests in survival. In both cases, patients may choose suicide and request assistance in its commission, but in one case they may do so for confused motives, and in the second case they may do so for motives not entirely their own because they have been subtly coerced.

The second criterion's requirement that suicidal motives be cogent turned out to be somewhat fragile, in that we seem to intuitively incline to overlook confused motives for doing the right thing. The third criterion's requirement that suicide not contravene interests has to be more robust. What we're looking at, then, is the relative weight of patients' value interests in survival with respect to their minimal or negative prudential interests in survival as determined by clinicians' expert assessment. Application of the third criterion has to do with protecting interests, and in medical contexts, that becomes a rather complex, dualistic matter because of the distinctions we drew among the various senses of "in one's interests." The main opposition here is between patients' value interests, or how patients value the life left to them, and patients' prudential interests, or how clinicians evaluate patients' interests in survival. Recall that prudential interests refers to a *communal* assessment of someone's stake in continued life. When clinicians assess patients' prudential interests as minimal or negative, they are judging that little or no justification is necessary for patients to relinquish life, or even that justification has become necessary to cling to life. The danger in all this is that suicide may be rendered irrational by contravention of value interests[28] even when prudential interests in survival are close to nil. Autonomy requires that individuals' lives be respected as theirs to retain or forfeit as *they* see fit.

Though others may judge that a given person's prudential interest in survival has evaporated because of an utterly hopeless prognosis, that doesn't suffice to compel that individual to commit suicide. All the good sense in the world, and the most reliable prognoses, aren't enough to warrant clinicians pressuring patients into assisted suicide—regardless of how compassionately. Choosing to die and committing suicide must be wholly autonomous acts, at least to the degree that any human action can be. The forfeiture of life by a rational agent must be that agent's own act. The criteria for rational suicide, though they involve the evaluative and informative participation of others, apply most directly to an agent's own autonomous decisions. Although others may contribute information and advice to an agent's decision regarding suicide, their contributions must stop short of significant influence, or autonomy will be jeopardized. In medical contexts, though, it is extremely difficult to draw, much less maintain, the distinction between the contributions of clinicians to suicidal deliberation and their significant influence. A hospitalized individual is highly vulnerable to influence, and those who are most likely to influence that individual are people regularly working with patients in hopeless situations in which life becomes a liability. The threat is that clinicians may too readily anticipate that end point and unduly discount patients' value *and* possibly prudential interests. Just as some patients may misperceive the time left to them as of no importance, clinicians may be prompted—perhaps quite unconsciously—by their experience and knowledge to influence patients' deliberations about their options in ways that inordinately tilt the balance toward suicide.

At present, clinicians tend to be conservative, perhaps too often working counterproductively to maintain life.[29] However, our concern is with what may result from the adoption of new attitudes. Aside from clinicians' training and professional values and priorities, they are affected by an inevitable measure of inurement to death and dying resulting from significant experience with terminal patients. That inurement may skew their perception of patient interests if assisted suicide comes to be accepted as a valid treatment option. We may find the familiar overestimation of patient interests quickly changing to systematic *under*estimation if clinicians train and work in an atmosphere of ready acceptance of assisted suicide. While overzealous efforts to keep some patients alive may result in greater suffering, it seems clear that underestimating patients' interests poses at least as great a danger.

Even when the danger of underestimation of patient interests is minimal, clinicians' solid determination of patients' prudential interests in survival may not be matched by their determination of patients' *value* interests. This failure may be due not to lack of expertise or sensitivity on the part of clinicians but to patients themselves being unclear about exactly what they want. It is precisely when patients are confused or ambivalent that the threat of undue influence is greatest and autonomy is most at risk.

The solution favored by many is to consider assisted suicide permissible only when someone is in so bad a condition that escaping it must be worth sacrificing the balance of life in anyone's judgment.[30] Suicidists clearly harm themselves in taking their own lives, because they deprive themselves utterly and irrevocably[31] of "pleasures, satisfactions, and other goods."[32] But there are times when it is evident to all that suicide does *less* harm than continuing to live, making self-destruction in one's interests. In these cases, the nature of anticipated experience has turned wholly negative, and life has ceased to be the condition of value and has become the enabling condition of disvalue, of suffering without adequate compensation. To kill oneself in these cases is to "deprive" oneself only of suffering. Provision of assisted suicide, then, seems permissible when suffering is hopeless, great enough, and evident.[33] At that point, patients' reasoning, motivation, and value interests are taken to be overridden by irremediable suffering and obvious loss of prudential interest in survival. In effect, the rationality of life's forfeiture is itself judged to be evident.

The picture painted is persuasive; it's a picture of clinicians compassionately helping patients to die when relinquishing life seems obviously to serve their best interests. It even may be felt, as we hinted earlier, that providing aid in dying in these circumstances is not only permissible but actually morally obligatory. However, there are two major difficulties with this picture. One is that it glosses the crucial difference between assisted suicide and voluntary euthanasia; the other is that it puts too much weight on clinicians' judgments.

Regarding the first difficulty, the fact is that the patients in the described cases aren't likely candidates for assisted suicide at all. Assisted suicide requires a certain measure of reflection and capability for action as a primary agent. If we take these extreme cases as central examples of assisted suicide, we run a serious risk of emptying the rationality requirement of content. The term *assisted suicide* would cover everything from helping coolly reflective and resolute but incapacitated individuals to take their lives, to putting persons no longer capable of rational thought out of their mind-destroying misery.

The importance of the difference between assisted suicide and voluntary euthanasia is basically that the more extreme patients' suffering is, the less likely that they can autonomously commit suicide. As suffering increases, patients' ability to reason clearly and to make sound decisions decreases proportionately. It's much more likely that patients suffering greatly will simply want to escape their torment and beg for death. Nonetheless, many clinicians construe these extreme cases as instances of suicide purely on the basis that the patient *wants* to die. But the matter is considerably more complex. The key point is that an expressed wish to die is not itself a self-destructive choice: *Wanting* to die need not be preparedness to kill oneself. Consider that a person prohibited by religious beliefs from committing suicide may want to die and *pray* for death but be wholly unwilling to take their own life. It matters whether patients are helped to commit suicide—i.e., helped to kill themselves—or are killed. If patients are suffering greatly and beg to die, perhaps the most humane thing to do is to kill them. But if they're killed, that doesn't mean they killed *themselves* by begging for death.

Many clinicians and some clinical ethicists think that there's no important distinction between assisted suicide and voluntary euthanasia. They focus, as noted, on the patient's desire not to live in the relevant circumstances. They assume that if the desire not to live is genuine, then the realization of that desire—i.e., whether the patient or a clinician causes death—is of secondary importance. Certainly it may be a matter of *practical* indifference whether we call some deaths assisted suicide or voluntary euthanasia. But from the theoretical perspective, the concern is about erosion of the primacy of agency in acts as significant as taking life. The long-term policy implications of describing voluntary euthanasia as assisted suicide could be extremely serious.

The theoretical worry can be clarified by considering a legal parallel. In the courts, particularly the criminal courts, fine but necessary distinctions are drawn between what someone did and what someone caused to be done by request, payment, or intimidation. Charges and penalties can be quite different in a case, depending on whether a defendant provided the means for another person to commit suicide or killed that person.[34] The basic point is that there *is* a line to be drawn between taking one's own life and having one's life taken, even if at one's own request. The proper paradigm for assisted suicide doesn't involve someone almost mindlessly begging for death; rather, it involves someone asking a physician to prescribe or provide some lethal dosage that the individual can take or not as they choose.[35]

The second difficulty, the weight given to clinicians' judgments, is that if we allow extreme suffering to transfer patients' autonomy regarding life-or-death decisions to clinicians, we invite problematic judgments by clinicians about patients' preparedness to end their lives. Consider the sort of aid in dying that is provided now, in some cases, regardless of illegality. Aid in dying is commonly provided—quite legally—as cessation of treatment. It is also provided, with patient or surrogate consent, by not treating certain conditions, such as pneumonia in severely demented patients. Patients are sedated and kept comfortable, but antibiotics aren't used, and the condition is allowed to run its course.[36] As noted earlier, this isn't described as passive euthanasia but as a judgment call about not prolonging dying with counterproductive treatment. What worries some theoreticians and slippery slope adherents is that this sort of compassionate judgment might begin to be made increasingly often, in less clear-cut cases, if assisted suicide becomes conventional and the term is too broadly applied to cases in which patients aren't primary agents.

The trouble is that third-party decisions about when someone's life no longer offers enough compensation for suffering, about when that someone loses prudential interest in survival, are determined by value-laden perceptions. This fact is offset to a degree by training and sensitivity, but that same training also conditions perceptions in a contrary way. The very expertise that enables clinicians to discern when patients have minimal or negative *prudential* interests in survival may inure clinicians to patients' *value* interests in survival. The result is that decisions about acceding to requests for assisted suicide may increasingly be made with insufficient attention to those value interests. This won't do, because for aid in dying to be assisted *suicide*, patients' value interests must play a decisive role both in their own decisions and in clinicians' decisions to provide assistance.

The important point regarding the third criterion and interests is that loss of prudential interest in survival isn't as conclusive a factor in decisions about assisting suicide as many take it to be. We are left, as in earlier chapters, with a question. We begin with patients whose prudential interests in survival are minimal or negative.[37] The matter of assisted suicide comes up in one or both of two ways: The likeliest is that patients express a wish to die; less likely but quite possible is that an attending clinician suggests or intimates that suicide should be considered as a way to avoid needless suffering. Once suicide arises as a possibility, and patients consider it as a Jamesian "living" option, our question has to do with how to best coordinate clinicians' provision of support for and assistance in suicide with patients' preparedness to die. The trick is ensuring that clinicians' perceived loss of patients' prudential interests in survival doesn't prompt unwarranted advocacy of suicide. Hasty or too eager provision of help or encouragement may contravene patients' autonomy through intimidation or simply by hurrying them.

A fairly tough-minded stand is that so long as there is a genuine desire to die on the part of patients, and patients' prudential interests are minimal or negative, it doesn't matter if patients remain somewhat ambivalent or are unready, because dying is what is best for them, and delaying can only result in greater suffering.[38] This view may be supported by appeal to human frailty in the sense that few manage complete resoluteness regarding their own death. But it *does* matter. It matters because we are at a point when we aren't just dealing with particular cases; we are determining policy regarding assisted suicide. Therefore, we must guard assiduously against establishing policies that erode personal autonomy.

A PREDICAMENT

Our central concern in this chapter is that interests not be contravened or unduly overridden in the provision of assistance in suicide. Once we sort out the important difference between value interests and prudential interests, it becomes clear that third-person judgments about prudential interests may conflict with first-person judgments about value interests. This is especially true of clinicians' judgments about patients' prudential interests. Clinicians have special and detailed knowledge of patients' conditions and prospects, which means that their more informed assessments can easily be at odds with patients' own assessments. Additionally, clinicians regularly engage in the assessment of prudential interests, whereas patients commonly have little experience

in doing so. We also have to add to the influences on clinicians' assessments the various institutional policies that bear on those assessments.
Assessment of prudential interests can be conducted on the basis of
public or "objective" information, such as test results and medical histories, whereas assessment of value interests involves problematic
probing of personal views and psychological states. This probing is often
inconclusive, because patients are fearful and feel vulnerable, sometimes becoming defensive and uncommunicative. Alternatively, they
may put on a brave but false front. Another complicating factor is an
increasing need for clinicians to adhere to cost-cutting policies, which,
among other things, means that they have less time to get to know their
patients. Value interests, then, pose an intractable problem with respect
to the permissibility of assisted suicide.

But however difficult to discern, in the main, patients' value interests should be decisive in the sense that, so long as we are considering
assisted suicide, a self-destructive decision must be autonomous to be
rational. This means that it must be made freely, knowingly, and resolutely, which in turn means that it must accord with patients' value
interests or, differently put, their value-laden perceptions of their prudential interests. But although clinicians and clinical ethicists agree that
patients' autonomous choices are primary, many are unconvinced that
there's as much real or potential conflict as suggested between patients'
choices and clinicians' decisions. The basis for this view is extensive
experience with actual cases, and what is usually emphasized is
patients' desire not to live under certain conditions.[39] In this view, a
patient's essential self-destructive act isn't performance of the physical
action of self-killing but is requesting assisted suicide or voluntary
euthanasia. Patients' high level of dependence, their desire to die, and
their requests for assistance in realizing that desire seem to put clinicians' accession to patients' requests comfortably into Beauchamp's
third category of "conditions arranged by the person for the purpose of
bringing about his or her own death."[40] Therefore, once a request for
assisted suicide is made, patients' value interests may be taken as manifest in the request.[41]

Again, we have a plausible picture; but again, we have a problem.
Earlier we proposed that the prudential interest in survival is, minimally,
the sum of the broadest-based considerations regarding the justification
of life's forfeiture. What this comes to is communal standards of what does
and doesn't warrant the willing abandonment of life. The problem is that
institutional medical establishments (i.e., hospitals, nursing homes, and
hospices) constitute communities, and the communal standards of those

establishments are not necessarily the same as those of the wider society. What counts as a significant prudential interest in survival in the wider society may not count as a significant interest in survival within a medical community. This means that assessment of patients' prudential interests may be significantly more negative within the medical community than outside it. Also, what counts as a significant or even decisive value interest in the wider society may be taken as overridden by minimal or negative prudential interests within a medical community.

Here we again see the gap between theory and practice. To the theorizing ethicist, it is of paramount importance to protect patient autonomy, and here autonomy has to do with value interests or what individuals perceive as their best interests. For the theoretician, then, the operant standards for assessment of prudential interests must be those of the wider community, because it is those standards that define rationality and hence reasonable valuation. But to the practicing clinician, the operant standards are usually those of the narrower expert community. From the perspective of clinicians, the wider community's standards are only of indirect relevance, because they are inexpert or uninformed. That is, those standards are seen as relevant only with respect to clinicians' accountability for treatment decisions, not with respect to the making of medical decisions.

It previously emerged that among the various pressing questions about assisted suicide, one of the most immediate is whether the proper focus for assessment of the rationality of suicide in medical contexts is patients' particular reasoning or their general competence. Another is about when patients' motives for wanting to die become immaterial to decisions about assisted suicide. It may have looked as if these questions should be answerable in terms of patients' interests. That is, once we sorted out the sense of "in one's interests" that is most relevant to the assisted suicide issue, we might have expected that questions about the focus of impairment assessment and the importance of motives would be resolved in terms of patients' prudential interests in survival. Roughly, it seems plausible that impairment assessment and evaluation of motivation would be largely determined by how much is at stake in consideration of assisted suicide.

However, in this chapter it's become clear that assessment of loss of prudential interest in survival isn't as decisive a factor as we might have thought. Contrary to what many believe, and to what we might have hoped, our questions aren't answered by recourse to loss or severe diminishment of prudential interest in survival. The reason is that third-party assessment of prudential interests as lost or negative[42] is rendered problematic by first-person value interests and how third persons' judgments are inevitably colored by their own priorities. We can't solve difficulties with assisted suicide in medical contexts by saying that suicidal reasoning, motives, and value interests become immaterial to the permissibility of assistance in commission of suicide when prudential interests are expertly judged minimal or negative. The very expertise that enables sound judgments about prudential interests impugns those judgments to a degree, because they may differ significantly from judgments made according to the standards of the wider community—which, of course, includes patients themselves.[43] If we resolve this predicament by giving special weight to clinicians' judgments because of their expertise and experience, we open the door to exactly what adherents of the slippery slope argument fear: application of special standards by a privileged group.

In the next chapter we finally come to grips with the slippery slope argument. While the foregoing chapters establish that suicide *can* be rational and that assisted suicide *can* be permissible, we seem to continually return to whether the criteria that determine that rationality and permissibility can be reliably applied in practical, clinical contexts.

SUMMARY

Rational suicide must benefit an individual more than continuing to live. This means that even if suicide appears to be an individual's best option and that individual chooses to commit suicide, doing so doesn't contravene the individual's prudential interests, as determined by broad communal standards, *and* the individual's value interests. But in medical contexts, the perception and assessment of potential suicidists' prudential interests in survival are always colored by clinicians' expertise, job-related experience, and priorities. The relative significance of patients' value interests may be seriously underestimated. What count as significant value interests in the wider community may be judged less so in professional contexts, and what count as significant prudential interests in survival in the wider community may not be deemed significant enough within those same professional contexts. The worse the prognosis, the easier it is to justify assisting suicide or making treatment decisions that may prejudice patients' prospects.[44] Bad enough prognoses also may move clinicians to directly or indirectly, knowingly or unknowingly, unduly influence patients' decisions. The consequence is that we can't rely on the apparent loss of prudential interest in survival to decide questions about the permissibility of assisted suicide. Flawed deliberation on the part of patients doesn't cease to matter, nor do confused motives become immaterial, when patients are judged to have lost their prudential interests in survival. This is because autonomy requires that their value interests be given due weight.

NOTES

1. The latter is the idea that if an individual's interest in survival is minimal or negative, that individual has no business clinging to life.

2. Rosenthal 1997, quoting Dr. Diane Meier, see also Kristol 1993.

3. Checkland and Silberfeld 1993:453.

4. See "Congress Weighs More Regulation on Managed Care," *New York Times*, March 10, 1997. The article addresses the question of HMO opposition to regulation and government's concern about protecting patients' options and treatment, asking, "If everybody backs patients' rights, why so much discord?" (sec. B, p. 8).

5. In the likeliest case, the decisions will be about how aggressively patients' conditions are treated. Physicians may decide not to treat pneumonia aggressively in the case of a terminal patient who, even though competent to give or withhold consent, is judged too near death to benefit from such treatment.

6. We aren't suggesting that there is deliberate duplicity here, but it's a fact that clinicians' own values and perceptions color how they deal with patients in these cases, regardless of professional, legal, and institutional requirements for full disclosure and consent.

7. It is important to keep in mind that suffering includes both physical pain and the range of psychological turmoil patients may experience, such as fear, loss of independence, loss of dignity, and so forth.

8. Even when someone is willing to bear great pain to achieve some goal, there are limits to what human beings should and can stand. See Hamel and DuBose 1996.

9. Patients in extremis, whose pain can no longer be relieved short of inducing unconsciousness, may well be beyond being able to think that it is in their best interests to bear their agony in the hope that their situations might improve.

10. Again, the sort of thing that has to be guarded against is patients requesting assisted suicide not because they choose to die but because they think that it is somehow expected of them or owed by them to those caring for and supporting them.

11. Since John Stuart Mill, utilitarians have acknowledged that the "optimific act," the act that does in fact have the best consequences, can't be required by the principle of utility (the moral directive to act to most benefit the greatest number). The reason is that requiring the optimific act would be to preclude moral action, since no one can know with certainty what act will in fact most benefit the greatest number.

12. We might observe that the playing field can't be leveled: Patients are and will remain dependent on clinicians, else they wouldn't be patients. We've avoided the contemporary trend to use euphemisms, such as calling patients "clients," in order not to obscure the simple fact that someone who is hospitalized, especially in a terminal situation, is dependent on attending clinicians. Patients' wishes and decisions ultimately can be respected only to a point. Changing terminology changes none of this.

13. For instance, unrealistic ideas about showing courage in the face of adversity may prompt one person to claim to want to die to prove their bravery but may prompt another person to deny wanting to die because of fear of appearing cowardly.

14. One difficulty with this fourth sort of case is evident in how supporters of assisted suicide tend to use only examples of the first and second cases, while detractors invariably rely most heavily on examples of the fourth.

15. It may be that voluntary euthanasia, or perhaps even involuntary euthanasia, is as easily justified in these cases.

16. This is, in the end, a subjective judgment, and it is extremely difficult to say who best decides what is or isn't bearable. But perhaps things aren't all that relative. We are, after all, actually pretty good at making these judgments. In addition, someone who has not experienced great pain before can be made to understand that higher levels of pain than they have had are in fact tolerable. This question of the degree to which subjective experience is wholly private is both an old philosophical one and one on which we are seriously at odds.

17. It's these latter cases that most worry theoreticians and advocates of the slippery slope argument, given the vulnerability of patients and the relative power of attending clinicians. But note that the point here is not whether the clinician's conviction that death is the wisest choice is or isn't a compassionate judgment; it very likely is just that. The point is that the patient's autonomy may be jeopardized by the clinician's influence.

18. That is, these are neither cases of suicide committed to escape immediate suffering nor cases of suicide committed in anticipation and well in advance of great suffering. Instead, these are cases of suicide in which patients are already suffering significantly and wish to avoid increased further suffering. See Prado 1990; Taylor 1995.

19. Reasons vary, of course, but the likeliest are religious convictions that any form of self-destruction is an unforgivable sin.

20. Of course, such judgments are not made without reluctance and ambivalence, given that what is at issue is someone's life.

21. The reasons here likely have to do with unwillingness to survive while hospitalized and dependent.

22. It might also be maintained that at this point patients are no longer capable of fully rational reflection because of contextual coercion.

23. See note 5 in chapter 3 on the incommensurability argument.

24. Battin 1984:312.

25. The senses of "in one's interests" discussed here are not exhaustive, but they do capture what is of greatest relevance to our project. Bond 1988:279.

26. This conflation results in a fourth sense of "in one's interests" that needs to be noted, because it's appealed to in arguments against the rationality of suicide. The idea here is that there is a sense, separate from the prudential, in which something is in our interests objectively, that is, regardless of perspective. Some contend that we all have an absolute interest in continued life, i.e., an objective or "real" interest in survival, because life is an irrevocable gift of God or part of an essential human nature. Interests in this objective sense, if there are any, would mostly be identical with prudential interests but would supersede anything deemed a prudential interest if that interest were not in fact an objective one—however that might be determined. This fourth sense is contentious, because many find it incoherent to speak of interests that are independent of the desires and perspectives of those whose interests they are supposed to be.

27. The question of improvement is a complex one, in that there could be improvement of the patient's condition, improvement of the patient's tolerance, or some combination of both.

28. Again, such contravention in the present discussion is taken to be undue influencing of patients' decisions or treatment decisions that in one way or another limit patients' options.

29. Malcolm 1990.

30. Note that restricting assisted suicide to these extreme cases wouldn't be a matter of keeping the status quo regarding the acceptance of assisted suicide, because as we've pointed out more than once, assisted suicide is presently provided, and it is provided in cases falling well short of the extreme in question.

31. To say this need not be to deny an afterlife in which value may be attained; it is only to say that earthly life as the condition of earthly value is irrevocable.

32. Battin 1984:308; Feinberg 1984:79–83.

33. Some think that there are cases when the sufficiency of suffering is evident to all, envisaging a hapless individual writhing in agony and having absolutely nothing to lose by forfeiting life to escape torment. There are cases like that, but we have to keep in mind that it is simply not the case that a sufficiency of suffering will always be evident and compelling to everyone concerned with a particular case.

34. Dr. Kevorkian's several trials illustrate the point. His "death machine" enables the people who have recourse to it to kill themselves, even if the appa-

ratus is set up for them. Dr. Kevorkian's intent is to provide the *means* for suicide, not to perform voluntary euthanasia.

35. Coutts and Hess 1996.

36. One of us heard a clinician describe the very high likelihood of pneumonia following an 87-year-old Alzheimer's patient's osteoporosis-related fracture as "a window of opportunity." The point being made was that the naturally occurring pneumonia provided a way of allowing the patient to die without anyone actually causing that prudentially advisable death.

37. There is an important difference. One person may have no further prudential interest in survival but be facing a tolerable death; another may have no further prudential interest in survival and have a prudential interest in dying to avoid an agonizing death.

38. At least one of us has heard this view expressed by a clinician on more than one occasion.

39. There is evidence, especially with cancer patients, that increased deterioration brings a heightened desire that attending physicians will perform voluntary euthanasia. Diegner and Sloan 1992.

40. Beauchamp 1980:77, quoted in Rachels 1986:81.

41. Many therefore think that all that needs to be determined, given the requests, is whether there are sound medical reasons to warrant patients' deaths—and that is to assess patients' prudential interests. Of course, it also needs to be determined whether patients' desire to die is genuine or the result of clinical depression or a similar preclusive condition.

42. The phrase "better off dead" seems to have no reliable third-person usage except when the individuals to whom it's applied are well beyond being capable of judging the phrase applicable in the first person.

43. A point made by a colleague, E. J. Bond, about concert reviews is, surprisingly enough, relevant here. The point was that reviews shouldn't necessarily be written by people who are expert in music, because their assessments are determined by an expertise not shared by members of typical audiences. Maria Callas once made a similar point, dismissing critics' assessments of her performances on the grounds that she sang "for the people." Old-enough readers of *The New Yorker* will recall the changes in film reviews by Pauline Kael after she spent some time in Hollywood, familiarizing herself with directors' problems and perspectives. There's something important in all this regarding the relevance of sets of standards that are, on the whole, mutually exclusive. Our predilection to value expert assessments more highly raises questions about precisely what standards are most applicable in particular cases.

44. For example, some potentially life-prolonging treatment might be deemed too "aggressive" in a case in which clinicians anticipate a request for assisted suicide.

6

THE SLIPPERY SLOPE

As has emerged, the determination that suicide in medical contexts is rational faces apparently intractable problems. We've focused on how application and satisfaction of three minimal theoretical requirements—our criteria for rational suicide—may be inadequate for various reasons. The reasons we've considered center on how clinicians' expertise, experience, and compassion, and their power relative to patients' vulnerability and dependency, may negatively affect the rationality and autonomy of patients' suicidal decisions. Diminishment of the rationality of suicidal decisions, and/or contravention of autonomy, means not only that suicide is jeopardized as a rational act but also that the permissibility of assisting suicide's commission is threatened or precluded. Specifically, the reasons why the criteria may be inadequately applied and met have to do with three possibilities: first, precipitous acceptance of patients' impaired suicidal reasoning; second, indifference to patients' confused motives; and third, neglect of patients' value interests through overreliance on diagnostic and prognostic assessments of patients' prudential interests in survival.

The foregoing problems admit of two contrary interpretations: They can be seen as calling for balance of theoretical and practical considerations, as we've proposed, or they can be seen as support for the slippery slope argument against the acceptance of assisted suicide as a sanctioned practice. There's good reason to see the problems as grist for the slippery slope mill. The questions we've considered are posed from a largely theoretical perspective, so they tend to take a darker view of possible profes-

123

sional trends. However well clinicians' provision of assistance in suicide may have worked in the past, and however well it may work in the future,[1] the theoretical concern must be with what is likeliest to go wrong if assisted suicide becomes a conventional treatment option.[2] What prompts our questions, then, is the worry that practicing clinicians may become increasingly less concerned with the niceties of determining the rationality of suicide once assisted suicide is a conventional option—whether or not formally legalized. But the reasons for concern about this possible outcome have little or nothing to do with paranoid fears that clinicians want to hurry their patients into self-destruction and are deterred only by illegality. The reasons have to do with how training, expertise, experience, authority, and compassion itself[3] shape and condition how clinicians perceive and appraise patients' situations and interests. The effect of these factors on clinicians' decisions is a hard fact,[4] and reflection on those factors can go only so far to mitigate their effect.[5] There's also no denying that there are new and serious pressures on clinicians to hold down the cost of caring for patients, and it would be naïve to think that these pressures don't affect treatment decisions at least some of the time.

We believe that the problems considered aren't intractable and are amenable to resolution through balanced application of theoretical and practical considerations. What we need to do, then, is to show how the mere persistence of these problems doesn't preclude the viability of assisted suicide as a sanctioned practice. That means showing that the slippery slope argument isn't a decisive bar to acceptance of assisted suicide. In other words, we need to show that the fact that there's an ever-present possibility that assisted suicide will be abused doesn't, of itself, disallow the practice. Basically, we think that the argument is usually misunderstood. It isn't an argument to establish the inevitability of certain undesirable possibilities; rather, it works as an ongoing constraint on abuse of assisted suicide. To make our case, we can begin by forming a clearer picture of the slippery slope debate. The following captures an important opposition that is too often obscured in claims and counter-claims about the dangers of the slippery slope:

> Virtually every major medical organization ... opposes physician-assisted suicide. ... But a few recent surveys have found that a majority of practicing doctors favor legalizing the practice and that, if it were legal, about a third of them would help patients commit suicide. ... In a recent survey of Michigan doctors, 56 percent said they supported allowing a doctor to help a patient commit suicide, and 35 percent said they "might offer" to help if it were legal. Sixty percent of

doctors in Oregon approve, another study found. A study of cancer specialists found that 57 percent had been asked for help in suicide and that 13.5 percent had written a lethal prescription. . . . [T]he divide between organized medicine and practicing doctors on the issue reflects . . . that medical groups are focused on the good of society while individual doctors have their patients in mind.[6]

What's important here is the contrast between medical groups and individual practitioners. The society-practitioner contrast is essentially a theory-practice one. Medical societies' concerns about the public good are the same as legal concerns about what will "flow from" legalization of assisted suicide for society at large, and both are of a piece with theoretical reservations about the proper governance of assisted suicide once it becomes a sanctioned practice.

"We've all had that patient who is in particularly dire straits where we might have gone that extra step to relieve their suffering, . . . [b]ut that is different than making public policy."[7] One of the most immediate causes for reluctance to make policy decisions supporting assisted suicide has to do with awareness of how well-intentioned legislation is often distorted and misused in practice.[8] Many clinicians worry that if assisted suicide becomes a conventional treatment option,[9] "managed-care companies trying to save money will pressure doctors to use this 'cost efficient' option." The fact is that *"suicide is cheap."*[10] The temptation could be to use suicide not as a *last* resort but as "the attractive solution of first resort."[11]

We just don't know how assisted suicide might be abused if it becomes a conventional treatment option, but the point here is the difference between attitudes toward individual clinicians providing assisted suicide and attitudes toward the provision of assisted suicide being institutionalized.[12] This point is at the heart of the slippery slope argument: We can't predict how assisted suicide, done by individuals in special circumstances, will turn out as a conventional practice once proscription is lifted and assisted suicide is acknowledged and sanctioned. As we've stressed, assisted suicide is done now, and it's a plausible view that we should leave well enough alone and trust the wisdom and discretion of compassionate clinicians.

The practice of medicine involves many judgment calls by clinicians. Regardless of ethical, legal, and professional regulations requiring patients' or surrogate decisionmakers' informed consent, there is a great deal of latitude in how judgment calls are made and communicated to patients, peers, and institutional authorities. This is recognized by clinicians and is one of the main reasons why "many doctors" want the provision of assistance in suicide to remain a purely medical matter. In that way, "willing doctors can continue to help desperate patients kill themselves quietly,"[13] without the repercussions attendant on social and professional acknowledgment and acceptance—and possible legalization—of the practice.[14] The trouble is, we aren't sure that things *are* well enough to leave alone. For one thing, "any medical practice that is surreptitious is hazardous, because it prevents review of documents and standards."[15] If the circumstances of assisted suicide cry out for individual, contextual procedures, its practice cries out for sound ethical and legal governance.

There's an undeniable, and no doubt healthy, distrust of institutionalization of assisted suicide, and that's what the slippery slope argument addresses. Basically, the fear is that once clinicians don't have to risk their careers and find ways to help patients die that can be legitimized under present regulations, provision of assisted suicide could become much too routine. As we've seen in the previous chapters, there are various ways in which this fear may be justified. Given the need to make a suicidal decision in a medical context, patients are vulnerable participants applying broad communal values and standards to a situation unique in their experience. Against this, clinicians are experienced, expert assessors applying professional and institutional values and standards to familiar situations. Lifting prohibitions could have unwelcome long-term effects.

Once we admit that there are clear dangers to accepting assisted suicide as a practice, the question arises whether those dangers are preclusive of acceptance of the practice or only call for great care in its governance. This is a pressing question, because regardless of obstacles to its legalization,[16] suicide and assisted suicide have gained a measure of societal plausibility that won't be easily dislodged. Attitudes are changing. Though suicide is condemned by Christianity, Judaism, and Islam, in recent years, the suicide rate among the elderly has risen 21 percent. The right-to-die movement is gaining strength, and the medical profession is shifting its traditionally conservative stand on the issue and seems more prepared to provide assistance in suicide.[17]

Resistance to these developments is a mix of moral, religious, professional, and sociopolitical claims. The resistance is articulated in various arguments, such as that life is sacred and that clinicians' obligations are to preserve life, not to take it. But as we noted at the outset, the most effective and widely supported argument against sanctioning assisted suicide is the slippery slope one. This argument accommodates diverse views, appealing mainly to the threat and consequences of systematic abuse.

With respect to the question of whether the dangers attendant on the practice of assisted suicide are preclusive, the slippery slope argument is almost invariably taken as maintaining that those dangers *are* preclusive, and that societal acceptance of assisted suicide will inexorably lead to the most vulnerable people being unwillingly "helped" to die.

What drives the slippery slope argument is a mix of realism, cynicism, and fear. As we pointed out earlier, historical precedents actually play a surprisingly secondary role in either making or countering the argument, which is essentially an expression of mistrust in our constancy to principle. The argument's adherents feel that we can't trust ourselves with sanctioned power over life and death. The basic assumption is that social acceptance of assisted suicide eventually would result in expediency usurping compassion in the treatment of the terminally ill, the very elderly, and the severely disabled. None who oppose acceptance believe for a moment that assisted suicide isn't presently done even where illegal. But the feeling is that to keep assisted suicide under control, it must remain socially interdicted and illegal. The expectation is that when assisted suicide is warranted in extreme cases, the courts will have the wisdom not to punish those who act compassionately though contrary to law. The thinking, then, is that what is endured by those who are charged with and tried for providing warranted assistance in suicide is a fair price to pay to protect ourselves from abuse of the practice.

The thrust of the slippery slope argument is that sanctioning assisted suicide will lead to people being killed against their will. But few adherents of the argument expect clinicians to start forcibly injecting their patients with potassium chloride.[18] "Against their will" has to be understood less literally to appreciate precisely what is feared. As we've stressed, the threat isn't outright prioritizing of expediency over humane treatment of patients considering suicide, but the diversity of perceptions that intersect in the making of decisions about the provision of assistance in suicide. And more important than the effects of particular perceptions is how they interact with one another and reshape themselves in the process of interaction. Psychiatrist Herbert Hendin captures what's crucial here by focusing on the complex and very particular personal and emotional dynamics of the individual cases in which assisted suicide is deliberated.[19] Hendin paints a picture of fluid situations in which many attitudinal forces interact and in which participants' differing conceptions of what is being considered often go undetected, even though contributing significantly to shaping decisions. Hendin's basic point is that we have no reliable means to control such situations. He believes that deliberations about assisted suicide can't be properly monitored, much less effectively regulated. The consequence is that regardless of the best intentions, ethical, professional, and even legal principles may be applied unevenly, misapplied, or ignored. In effect, Hendin generalizes our concerns about the application of the criteria for rational suicide to the application of all relevant standards. In Hendin's view, social acceptance of assisted suicide would sanction a practice based on uncontrollable considerations; it would open the door to widespread disparity in treatment of potential suicidists and to the possibility of serious abuse.

Charles Rosenberg succinctly summarizes Hendin's point as follows: "The linked system of clinician, patient, family and friends is the focus of [Hendin's] argument—and he contends that the emotional dynamics will inevitably determine individual outcomes. The patient is often depressed . . . , relatives are guilt ridden and ambivalent, the physician is often driven by a need for closure and control when available technical tools are no longer relevant."[20] The concern is that given the "delicately balanced emotional and social system" that Hendin describes, assisted suicide's becoming a conventional option "would necessarily shape a new gradient in decision-making—steepening the incline of innumerable slippery slides toward premature death."[21]

It is this "steepening" of the inclination to use assisted suicide as a treatment option that the slippery slope argument warns against. And in doing so, it coincides with our concern that routine, added to unavoidable practical difficulties, may seriously degrade provision of assisted suicide. Pointed authoritative advice,[22] contextual constraints,[23] and inadequately disclosed treatment decisions[24] can force vulnerable patients into committing suicide. Even when patients avow their intentions to commit suicide, those who are despondent[25] or intimidated or otherwise suggestible may be hurried into self-destruction. If the prohibition against assisting suicide were removed, we could well find clinicians increasingly inclined to unduly influence terminal, elderly, and severely disabled patients to take their lives.

We might put things in this way: The slippery slope argument claims that once assisted suicide becomes a conventional alternative to letting a terminal illness run its course, to enduring hopeless disability, or to coping with debilitating advanced age, then that alternative is bound to be used. That much could be acceptable enough. With removal of the prohibition against assisted suicide, we could expect that many patients who are presently denied *warranted* assistance in self-destruction would receive it. The unacceptable part comes when we add increasingly scarce human and financial resources to the availability of the option, because then use may become abuse. The easiest—and subtlest—way that that happens is when expediency conveniently exaggerates compassion, in the sense that clinicians grow too ready to think that patients are better off dead than enduring their afflictions. At that point, the compassion that previously would have manifested itself in such actions as more aggressive sedation could manifest itself in disproportionate encouragement of self-destruction and easy accession to questionable requests for assistance in suicide.

"TRUST ME, I'M A DOCTOR"

The slippery slope argument is often dismissed by clinicians as prompted by ignorance and diffuse fear.[26] Clinicians fail to understand how anyone could suspect them of expediency-driven indifference, much less of malice or devious motives, toward people who are put in their care and for whom they're professionally responsible.[27] Alternatively, clinicians may see the slippery slope argument as thinly disguised intractable moral or religious opposition to assisted suicide, comparable to close-minded attacks on abortion. In this view, the argument is little more that a scare tactic prompted by refusal to consider seriously the sound medical reasons for the provision of assisted suicide.

The less reflective versions of the slippery slope argument may merit dismissal, but as we've suggested, its more thoughtful versions pose a challenge worthy of careful consideration. To clarify that challenge, the argument needs to be articulated not in the dramatic terms of the inevitability of sanctioned medical murder but in terms of a possibly preclusive imbalance of risk and gain in the establishment of assisted suicide as a sanctioned practice.

As we've stressed, one need not see hidden agendas in clinicians' treatment of terminal, very elderly, and severely disabled patients to feel genuine concern that those patients' interests may be unduly diminished in the complex process of evaluating prognoses and determining appropriate treatment.[28] One need understand only three elements that inevitably color clinicians' attitudes and the treatment decisions they make regarding patients in these categories: the inuring or at least tempering effect on clinicians of dealing with death on a professional basis; the vast difference between contemplating one's own or a loved one's death and contemplating a relative stranger's death; and contemporary budgetary pressures. It is not implausible to claim that a combination of these elements could make a significant difference—contrary to patient interests—in the weighing of negative prognostic factors when making both treatment decisions and decisions about the provision of assistance in suicide.

There is, in addition, a complicating factor: Budgetary pressures are not a simple matter of insufficient funds to pursue certain treatment options. Lack of funds and increasing costs have led to the adoption of a whole new perspective on health care. Dealing with health problems in our society has been recast from something like a care model to a business model. We hear a great deal about "managed care" and the "business paradigm." The underlying idea is that if health care is run on a market model, it will be more efficient and cost-conscious. This is the same idea we've seen working in our society's inclination to privatize services traditionally provided by governments. The trouble is that when patients become "clients," a fundamental caring element is eroded, if not lost. When hospital stays are dictated by accountants, when physicians can't suggest too-costly treatments to patients, when nurses are burdened with counting gauze pads, a gap opens up between clinicians and patients that is difficult to bridge.[29] The reason is that the patient ceases to be seen as a person to be cared for and comes to be seen, at bottom, as a *liability*.

The point is that adoption of the business model turns patients into consumers. But unlike consumers in a shop, patients in a hospital aren't paying enough and *can't* pay enough for the costly goods and services they consume. One way of encapsulating the effect of the business model is to say that part of the trust people had in physicians, nurses, and other health-care professionals was due to the assumption that they were in control of treatment, and that their motivation was altruistic. In fact, that kind of trust often led to patients being *too* trusting. But now clinicians aren't in control; others oversee many of their decisions, and the motives of those others are not altruistic. Regardless of rhetoric and political emphasis on fairer distribution and more efficient use of tax revenue, what drives the business model of health care is essentially mercenary;[30] otherwise, it's unclear why it's a *business* model or paradigm.

Some clinicians will respond that what's really happening is that we're now weighting prognostic factors more realistically than before, and that there is only a surface appearance of more expedient treatment decisions being made. However, it can also be claimed that expediency has begun to usurp compassion. While it is true that the medical tradition has been strongly oriented toward maintaining life at too great a cost to both patients and institutions, it does seem rather suggestive that we're experiencing a sea change in attitude toward the maintenance of precarious life just when North America's population is aging rapidly and making increasingly costly demands on the health-care system.[31]

If we put the point of the slippery slope argument neutrally, it's just that societal acceptance—and possible legalization—of assisted suicide will result in more assisted deaths. The fear underlying this point is that the increase won't be in warranted deaths, but rather that more deaths will occur because of expediency. However, the moment we specify the people most at risk, according to the argument, we see the other side of the issue and better appreciate the point about more realistic weighing of prognoses in treatment decisions. It's arguable that the terminally ill, the seriously debilitated elderly, and the severely disabled simply don't have a great enough prudential interest in survival to justify the efforts presently made to keep them alive. In other words, we have to factor into the equation the idea that in the past, too many people with little or no prudential interest in survival were kept alive in ways that actually contravened their well-being. If that idea is accepted, then the higher incidence of assisted suicides predicted by the slippery slope argument emerges as a justified rather than disturbing consequence of sanctioning assisted suicide. This, in effect, suggests that the slippery slope argument tends to confuse two quite different things: social and professional acceptance of assisted suicide resulting in a greater number of unwarranted deaths that *contravene* patients' interests, and acceptance resulting in a greater number of warranted deaths that *serve* patients' interests.

The suggestion that even a considerable increase in the number of assisted suicides might be warranted by better recognition and acknowledgment of loss of prudential interests in survival brings us to a key point regarding trust. If what is at issue is prudential interests in survival, then we need to be able to rely on clinicians to be scrupulous in keeping the assessment of prudential interests as free of skewing by practical, institutional, and personal considerations as is humanly possible. This means that those assessments mustn't be overly conditioned by clinicians' professional and personal views regarding human life. Unfortunately, determinations about the relative weight given to positive and negative factors in these assessments can't be made according to exact rules; in the end, the clinicians making the judgments are people whose professional assessments are inexorably influenced by a complex background of experience, training, and philosophical outlook, as well as institutional and practical pressures. The only recourse here is *con-*

sultation. Just as the role of others is crucial to ensuring the rationality of potential suicidists' deliberations, the role of consultants is vital to the safeguarding of patients' interests.[32]

Here again, the parallel with juries is helpful. Prosecutors and defense attorneys strive to impanel juries that will favor their respective sides. Providing advice on jury selection is now a sophisticated and apparently reliable business, and what it trades on is the reasonable predictability of how individuals of certain backgrounds will assess certain situations. If we thought of medical consultative groups dealing with decisions about assisted suicide as being somewhat like juries, we would want to exclude those who, because of training, experience, and philosophical inclination, would be too likely to reject the provision of assisted suicide. We also would like to exclude those who would lean too much toward expedient measures regarding the cost and effort of maintaining life. Since we can't achieve either of these objectives beyond a limited extent, what we want is a good mix of divergent perspectives to ensure that no one point of view dominates for lack of challenge. However, no matter how effective the consultative process, participants can address only the aspects of cases that are public: test results, medical histories, expert opinions, and so forth. This means that the focus remains on the assessment of prudential interests. Unfortunately, those interests are only half the story.

We can close this section by summarizing the foregoing points in this way: Whatever its merits or excesses, the slippery slope argument raises an important issue. Clinicians can be expected to make prognostic and treatment judgments and assessments in line with their experience, values, and degree of inurement to death and dying. Additionally, their judgments and assessments may be more or less influenced by technically extraneous matters such as budgetary considerations, caseloads, and institutional policies. Perhaps the most important influence on clinicians at present, and in the near future, is adoption of the business model of health care in both medical training and practice. Given these realities, there is a marked likelihood that if assisted suicide becomes an available treatment option, it will be used significantly more than at present. This isn't to say that suicidal decisions will be imposed on patients; it's to say that there will be greater and somewhat easier accession to requests for assisted suicide and probably more initiation by clinicians of consideration of assisted suicide. Some of the increase in assisted suicide will be warranted by patients' conditions and prognoses, but there is a danger that another part of the increase will be a function of various extraneous factors and pressures that contravene patients' interests to some extent.[33] Consultation among clinicians seems to be the obvious check on the possible abuse of assisted suicide, but such consultation naturally centers on patients' prudential interests in survival. However, it isn't only those interests that must be safeguarded against contravention, and it isn't only those interests—or rather their absence or negative nature—that warrant assistance in the commission of suicide.

THE SUBJECTIVE ELEMENT

If we had to contend only with prudential interests, the slippery slope argument, or at least the cautionary version outlined in the last section, would pose a much less serious challenge than it actually does. The reason is that from the perspective of the patient, prudential interests in survival, or prudential interests in dying, may be quite contrary to their *value* interests. Patients in utterly hopeless situations may not want to die; they may be willing to tolerate even great pain for whatever time is left to them. We also can imagine someone's moral or religious values barring them from taking what they might perceive as "the easy way out." Unless we are prepared to kill people for their own good, for what the community sees as their own best prudential interests, we must respect even what may appear to be profoundly foolish decisions to live on.[34] When we are dealing with human lives, and so long as we respect the principle of autonomy, we can't make life-or-death decisions purely on the basis of prudential interests. Even if those interests could be determined conclusively, and they obviously can't, they wouldn't suffice to warrant disregard for people's preferences regarding their own lives.

It may appear that these considerations don't apply here, since what concerns us is assisted suicide and thus an expressed desire to die on the part of the patients in question. But things simply aren't that clear-cut. Beside having to contend with expressed desires to die that could be products of undue influence or even manipulation, there are other important possibilities. Although associated with the mistaken view that suicide is always pathological, the idea that threatened suicide may be a cry for help is far from wrong. Expressions of a wish to die may be no more than indirect requests for reassurance or even sympathy. Usually resolute references to suicide can be fairly readily distinguished from avowals and requests that are driven by other motives, but this isn't always so. The difficult cases are when expressions of a wish to die fall somewhere between these extremes. Moreover, patients may declare that they want to die in what sounds like a resolute manner but is in fact a simulation of resolution covering deep ambivalence. Resolute-sounding declarations may serve less to inform others of a firm desire to die than to try to decide the issue in the patients' own minds. In any of these eventualities, to proceed on the basis that an expressed desire to die can be taken at face value could be to force patients into positions in which false pride or intimidation makes them kill themselves without wanting to.

It would be unacceptable to take the mere request by a patient for assisted suicide, together with a negative prognosis, as adequate warrant to provide assistance in the commission of suicide. This is where the danger is greatest that what Hendin describes as clinicians' desire for closure may result in coerced self-destruction. We would then have the nightmarish scenario feared by most slippery slope adherents: Someone's ill-considered request for assisted suicide is hastily acceded to, and the person is compelled by circumstances to commit suicide. And the act could still be *suicide*. That is, it needn't be some form of euthanasia, much less murder. The whole point is that patients in vulnerable positions can be made to do things they don't really want to do. The difference is that suicide in such cases, while still *self*-killing, would not be an autonomous act because of undue influence or contextual coercion. This is what has to be taken seriously in the slippery slope argument—that people can be maneuvered into self-destruction that is less than autonomous but is still their own action.

The questions raised by the slippery slope argument are neither met nor deflected by expressed desires to die. Those expressions are no more than a starting point for assessment. The concern about contravening value interests applies to assisted suicide so long as we lack a fail-safe way to determine the genuineness of expressed desires to die and the autonomy of resulting actions. The likeliest slide down the slippery slope isn't going from providing compassionate aid in dying to committing expedient murder. The likeliest slide is from the present possibly too cautious provision of aid in dying to overly brisk provision, based on assumptions that those with little or no prudential interest in survival themselves really want to die.[35]

Assisted suicide in medical contexts doesn't immediately raise the issue of outright violation of patient autonomy, as would involuntary euthanasia. It poses a question about erosion of autonomy through diminution of patients' value interests. The central point about that diminution is that it may come about not through overt changes in communal consensus on values and priorities regarding life-or-death decisions[36] but through individual clinicians' actions and tacit collegial complicity. In other words, rather than that diminution reflecting broad communal reconception of the weight that value interests merit, and adjustment of societal standards regarding respect for value interests, it will reflect only changes within a professional community.[37] The likeliest erosion of patient autonomy within the medical community will come about by reducing the importance of the subjective aspect of patients' consideration of suicide relative to prognostic and institutional priorities. The likeliest manifestation of that reduction will be insouciant acceptance of declarations of a desire to die when those declarations are in line with patients' conditions and prospects.

We might sum up the subjective aspect in this way: Distinguishing among the senses of "in one's interests" has as its primary point the contrast between what is in someone's interests because it's valued and wanted and what is communally judged to be in someone's interests, irrespective of what that person wants or values. Generally, if something is an interest generated by a desire, it may or may not be good for one. Third parties may be in a position to better understand what is in fact in someone's interests. In the case of someone considering suicide in a medical context, clinicians' experience, expertise, and detailed diagnostic and prognostic knowledge put them in a position to better understand a patient's prudential interests. In most cases, regarding anything from medication to major surgery, we are impatient with people who oppose clinicians' considered advice. But in the case of self-destruction, we have to be more careful. Someone's ambivalence about suicide may make little sense to us in certain circumstances, but unlike medication or surgery, what is at issue is not undergoing some potentially risky treatment or procedure for the sake of enhancing or preserving life, but deciding whether or not to end life. If we respect the fundamental Hippocratic principle of above all doing no harm, we can't contravene value interests, even if they are present only as indecision.[38]

What can put self-destruction on the side of benefiting rather than harming a patient is if it would spare the person in question needless suffering without contravening a significant prudential interest in survival. This occurs when, all things considered, it is in a person's interest to die because he or she has a minimal prudential interest in survival—e.g., is in a terminal condition or of greatly advanced age—compounded by anticipated irremediable suffering. This combination in effect means that the person has a negative prudential interest in survival, so a positive prudential interest in dying. But even given this combination, forfeiting life is still the affected individual's choice, no one else's. Exceptional value interests may alter the equation, for instance, deeply held religious beliefs that prohibit self-destruction or euthanasia. The exceptions, when value interests may be overridden, aren't relevant here, because they aren't cases of assisted suicide; they are cases of merciful euthanasia performed on individuals no longer capable of sound reasoning and/or unable to request or oppose aid in dying.

The crux of the slippery slope argument for us, then, is the danger that patients' minimal or negative prudential interests will be used to warrant discounting or even ignoring their value interests. When the matter of ending life is initiated by the patient, the danger posed by assisted suicide as a conventional treatment option takes the form of ambivalent, ill-considered, or confused suicidal decisions being insouciantly accepted by attending clinicians because of prognostic assessments and other pressures. In other words, the danger is inadequate application of the criteria for rational suicide because of undue weight given to negative appraisals of patients' prudential interests and corresponding underestimation of their value interests. What makes things difficult is that in the troublesome cases there will often be adequate, if not abundant, medical reasons to discount patients' perceptions of their own situations.

The slippery slope in cases of assisted suicide in medical contexts, then, is the possibility that societal and professional acceptance of assisted suicide, and its becoming a conventional treatment option, will foster hurried accession to questionable requests for assisted suicide, and especially that it will encourage undue influences on patients. These developments aren't anticipated as resulting from clinicians suddenly becoming brutally pragmatic about the cost of sustaining tenuous life, but as a consequence of changed perceptions, institutional exigencies, and imposition of the business model on health care.

A PENDING QUESTION

As we considered in chapter 1, the slippery slope argument is quite resistant to historical counterarguments. The Netherlands's apparent success[39] with condoned assisted suicide[40] and Australia's truncated experience with new legislation[41] are basically immaterial to the slippery slope argument at the present time. The argument doesn't contend that historical experience *establishes* that sanctioned assisted suicide has in fact resulted in abuse; its point isn't that past experience shows that abuse is inevitable. This is only in part because there's very little historical evidence, and we don't have enough to support *or* rebut that claim. The argument's real claim is that we will *create* an abusive practice by condoning assisted suicide as a medical practice. The argument's point is that we'll be initiating a practice, and fostering attendant perspectives, that will eventually devalue the lives of those who are seriously ill, greatly disabled, or simply very old. The worry behind the slippery slope argument has to do with the consequences of reeducating our society to countenance assisted suicide as an acceptable medical response to catastrophic illness and extreme debility.

The popular view is still that human life is of paramount importance, hence clinicians[42] are seen as mandated to do all in their power to save and sustain life. Anything short of diligent efforts to preserve life prompts communal outrage because it's perceived as a violation of that mandate. But now we've seen health maintenance organizations (HMOs) attempt to make even so traumatic an operation as mastectomy an outpatient procedure in order to trim costs.[43] We've also seen dramatic shifts in treatment priorities, a notable example being how access to liver transplants has changed from giving precedence to patients most in need to giving precedence to those most likely to benefit from the availability of organs.[44] The fact that assisted suicide in medical contexts is now hotly debated confirms that there is a sea change taking place in the conception of health care.

In remarks made in an interview on assisted suicide, Arthur Caplan captures the fears of many about

> an aging population that's going to be drawing down resources. People think now they're facing a system that's trying to ration. That is a mere hint of what is to come. . . . I worry that assisted suicide is not going to be the option of last resort—it's going to be the attractive solution of first resort. Not that we're going to have a government dictating, you must die, [but] that suddenly within the society, the notion will come that the older and disabled who are expensive should do the responsible thing.[45]

Caplan's reference to the old and disabled doing "the responsible thing" is precisely what is central to changing conceptions of health care and life maintenance. We may be undergoing a radical change in our attitude toward life and its maintenance, adopting an attitude that expresses new expectations of responsibility to younger, more able people in a society in which an aging population is increasingly pressuring the health-care system. These expectations will produce very different behavior on the part of both those requiring and those providing medical care. From our present communal perspective, we reject old customs such as elderly Inuit people walking away into the frozen wilderness when they can no longer contribute to their families. But from other perspectives, those are fitting and honorable customs. Older and dependent members of our society won't be going off into the wilderness any time soon, but they may have to accept minimal health care beyond a certain point in age, illness, and debility. One harbinger of things to come is HMOs in the United States limiting elderly patients' appeals of adverse decisions regarding access to certain forms of treatment.[46] The choice will be to endure slow death, unassisted by technology or even expert caregivers, or to commit suicide. Most adherents of the slippery slope argument see such developments as monstrous, but loss of care in highly dependent states is, in effect, more a loss of headway made than new denial. It's like a return to a time when it wasn't the *cost* of modern health care that prevented prolonging lives but its nonexistence. It's like a return to a time when death was a family burden rather than an institutional one.

Barring miraculous technological and economic breakthroughs, we probably have little choice about where we're heading as a society with respect to health care. Historically speaking, the era of life's prolongation with elaborate technology such as dialysis machines and ventilators has been brief. It is only within the past half-dozen decades that ordinary people with certain illnesses or disabilities could count on living well beyond the time their parents could have hoped to live with the same afflictions. To many contemporaries, it may appear that technologically prolonged life is a right, but it is hardly that. It is a privilege bestowed on its members by an affluent society. When society can no longer afford that largesse, it has to ration, as it has begun to do.

In light of present realities, the slippery slope argument will prove insufficient to preclude societal and professional—and possibly legal— acceptance of assisted suicide. But the argument shouldn't be dismissed; instead, it should be understood as a caution about the dangers of sanctioning the practice it opposes, and thus as a check on that practice. Seen in this light, the argument is a balancing tactic and calls not for rebuttal but for appreciation. Although this may be a propitious understanding of what initially looks like a preclusive obstacle to the acceptance of assisted suicide, it doesn't resolve our concerns about the misuse or abuse of assisted suicide in medical contexts. Problems persist about undue influence on patients and maintaining an equilibrium of patients' prudential and value interests. If a sea change is taking place in our view of health care and life maintenance, we must ensure that when decisions are made about the provision of assistance in suicide, clinicians'[47] assessments of patients' prudential interests don't systematically override confused reasoning, questionable motives, and value interests.[48]

To end this chapter, we need to put the foregoing remarks about the slippery slope argument in the context of the opposition between theoreticians and clinicians on the interpretation and application of our criteria for rational suicide.

It's worth reiterating that the criteria are offered as minimal theoretical requirements to determine whether something is an instance of rational suicide—i.e., an act of self-destruction that is the best available means to best serve the agent's values and interests. If an act of self-destruction is rational in the sense we've outlined, then it is permissible to assist its commission. Disagreements begin with how stringently the criteria are to be interpreted and applied, and so how accommodating they can be in permitting assisted suicide despite residual questions about reasoning, motives, and/or value interests.[49] So far, we've sketched a contrast between theoreticians' strict interpretation and application of the criteria and clinicians'[50] more forgiving contextual understanding and use of the criteria. With respect to reasoning, the split is over whether the criteria apply primarily to an individual's particular line of reasoning about self-destruction or to that person's general competence. With respect to motivation, the split is over the point at which a patient's particular motives are made immaterial by that person's actual and anticipated suffering. With respect to interests, the split is over when minimal or negative prudential interests override contrary value interests and allow clinicians to influence patients' decisions to some degree or to readily accede to requests for assisted suicide. We can now restate these differences in a more concise way in terms of default assumptions.[51]

For theoreticians, the default assumption is that there most likely will be flawed reasoning, faulty motivation, or misperception of interests in suicidal deliberation. This is not the common view that considering suicide is always pathological; it is recognition that deciding to end one's life, particularly because of an ominous medical condition, is rarely a coolly reflective and emotionally neutral exercise. Instead, it is a hugely stressful exercise full of irresoluteness and conflicting emotions. People under such stress face serious obstacles to clear thinking; their "judgment about probabilities may be seriously affected," and they may overemphasize the likelihood of negative events, "subconsciously suppressing data which lead to a more optimistic prediction."[52] Nor is it only perceptions of the future that are distorted. Not only do "good things in the future tend to seem less significant than bad things occurring now," but perceptions of the past are also affected because great stress and fear may "warp our recollections about our preferences."[53] This means that long-held values and priorities may not be allowed to play their proper role in suicidal deliberation. Ideals that have guided a person's lifelong choices and objectives may suddenly look empty and pointless and be eclipsed by unstable emotional responses and inclinations of the moment. To all these factors we have to add the complex influences and roles of others involved in Hendin's "linked system of clinician, patient, family and friends."[54]

Theoreticians see the exigencies that make people consider suicide as likely forcing or skewing choices that need to be made most carefully. That's why theoreticians think that suicidal deliberation should be approached as suspect. It's not that they think that wanting to die is crazy. They understand that the choice isn't one of death over life but is a matter of being unwilling to live under certain conditions. But those very conditions may distort deliberation and generate confused reasons for choosing not to live, thereby coercing individuals to make irrational choices. Therefore, the criteria for rational suicide need to be scrupulously applied to ensure that the decision made is the most rational that can be made in the circumstances.

Clinicians certainly agree that there is little cool reflection or emotional neutrality in the turmoil of suicidal deliberation, but their response isn't to increase the stringency of the demand for cogency in reasoning and motivation but to *decrease* it. Their inclination is to qualify or lessen the significance of reasoning errors and problematic motives in requests for assisted suicide. Clinicians are moved by the exigencies of terminal conditions to be more compassionately forgiving of patients' ambivalence and confusion. Clinicians' default assumption is that the weaknesses in patients' deliberations are of secondary importance to the desire to die, because the real warrant for self-destruction is provided not by those deliberations but by patients' medical conditions and prospects. If patients' suicidal deliberations are textbook exercises in sound reasoning, so much the better, but a fair bit less is acceptable if there are good medical reasons for self-destruction.[55]

It would appear that the very factors that make theoreticians worry that potential suicidists may be making errant self-destructive choices tend to incline clinicians to be more accepting of those choices. Whereas theoretical distance makes great suffering and dire prognoses good reasons to suspect confused deliberation about self-destruction, clinical involvement makes great suffering and dire prognoses good reasons to overlook confused deliberation about self-destruction. Put in different terms, when it comes to assessing requests for assisted suicide, theoreticians' commitment to abstract rationality prompts them to try to separate proffered reasons for suicide from the individual patient's punishing situation. In contrast, clinicians' practical experience prompts them to understand proffered reasons in the context of that punishing situation.

We can now reformulate the issue that the slippery slope argument raises in this way: First, we reconstrue the force of the argument not as precluding social and professional acceptance of assisted suicide but as counterbalancing the dangers of an admittedly risky practice. The heart of the argument is that compassionate aid in dying may turn into expedient influencing and hurrying of self-destruction if assisted suicide becomes a conventional medical practice. If we recast this point as an ongoing warning rather than a preclusive objection, we can see its value as a safeguard against abuse of assisted suicide. The thrust of the argument then becomes that opposition to assisted suicide should remain constant and current as protection against abuse.[56] Whatever their own intentions, adherents of the slippery slope argument serve to keep supporters and practitioners of sanctioned assisted suicide aware of the dangers that the practice entails. Second, the split between theoreticians and clinicians[57] can also be recast as one of balancing tactics. Theoreticians may be seen as employing their distance from practice to maintain an objective-observer perspective on what goes on in the provision of assisted suicide. Clinicians may be seen as employing their compassionate and empathic involvement with potential suicidists to check overly stringent theoretical demands. The effect is to preserve the gravity of decisions to assist the commission of suicide and to prevent provision of that assistance from deteriorating into disinterested routine.

As we noted at the outset, the most important parallel between assisted suicide and abortion is that both debates will remain unresolved because the opposed positions arise from a clash of profoundly divergent conceptions of human life. It is highly unlikely that one or the other of the two sides in either debate will be converted or that either of the debates will evaporate. As we've said, the most we can hope for is compromise and balance. It now looks as if those who think that life may be forfeited in certain circumstances will prevail in North America, as did those who think that women have the right to terminate unwanted pregnancies. The value of the slippery slope argument in these changed circumstances, then, should be seen not as a failed attempt to block acceptance of assisted suicide as a practice but as a constant reminder of its dangers.

SUMMARY

The slippery slope argument against societal and professional acceptance—and possible legalization—of assisted suicide initially poses an obstacle nearly as formidable as the claim that suicide is irrational. The argument maintains that assisted suicide will be abused and that rare, compassionate aid in dying will turn into common, expedient liquidation of the terminally ill, the severely disabled, and the very elderly. The argument tries to establish that, whatever the merits of assisted suicide in particular cases, what would flow from its acceptance for society at large is harmful. The argument appears to be an empirical one, suggesting an evidential base and vulnerability to counterexamples. But if we look more closely, we realize that historical and contemporary experience with legal assisted suicide, meager though it is, actually is immaterial to the slippery slope argument. The argument's real force has to do with the cumulative effects of adopting new attitudes toward life maintenance and how those attitudes will shape medical education and future medical practice. We've focused on how clinicians' assessments of patients' *prudential* interests in survival tend to underestimate the importance of patients' *value* interests. The real possibility of a slide down the slippery slope has little to do with clinicians' having hidden agendas, much less ill will toward their patients. It mainly has to do with how their assessments of patients' interests are based on the standards of a professional community—standards that may differ significantly from those of the wider community.[58] Once we understand this, the slippery slope argument's significance emerges as a persistent caution against allowing the permissibility of assisted suicide, in medical contexts, to become too much a function of professional and institutional evaluation of patients' interests.

NOTES

1. There's an interesting semantic point here that has dogged our steps throughout. Like most others concerned with the topic, and certainly the media, we have spoken of *provision of assisted suicide*. It's perfectly clear that what is provided is assistance *in the commission* of suicide, but it's easy to slip into hearing and reading the phrase as if it is assisted suicide that is provided, as euthanasia is provided. It's a subtle difference in meaning, but the latter understanding diminishes the role of the patient, the suicidist, by making it appear that assisted suicide is something that patients request and is *administered*, as any other treatment would be.

2. Ethical theory is, of course, primarily concerned with determining the acceptability of suicide and assisted suicide. But having offered criteria for when suicide—and, by extension, assisted suicide—*is* acceptable, our theoretical priority is a "defensive" one; the primary concern is that suicide *remain* acceptable despite practical difficulties.

3. Compassion is a fragile thing, and its force and character may vary considerably with experience. Someone inured to death and dying may well feel a different sort of compassion for suffering patients than someone having little experience with terminal illness. When a person having little experience with the dying is moved to offer greater care, an experienced individual will be moved to help end the suffering.

4. There's no question that individual clinicians may be quite successful at checking the effect of these factors in dealing with particular patients, but the point has to do with overall trends in the profession.

5. It's not even clear that their effect *should* be lessened by much, given that the factors in question are precisely those that enable well-informed medical decisions and have historically lent clinicians the authority that their patients respect.

6. Rosenthal 1997.

7. Rosenthal 1997.

8. "Zero tolerance" policies adopted in the schools, for instance, have had to be revised after cases such as the now infamous one of a six-year-old first-grader being suspended for sexual harassment for kissing a female classmate on the cheek (Lewin 1997).

9. Rosenthal 1997.

10. Battin 1987:169, emphasis in original. See also Bayer et al. 1983.

11. Interview with Arthur Caplan, "The Kevorkian Verdict," *Frontline*, broadcast May 14, 1996.

12. It's important to keep in mind that professional and societal acceptance of assisted suicide as a practice needn't require formal legalization.

13. Rosenthal 1997.

14. It's striking that "[m]any doctors who support the practice [of assisted suicide] in theory say they could not do it themselves" (Rosenthal 1997).

15. Rosenthal 1997.

16. For instance, the Clinton administration has gone on record as opposing assisted suicide (Greenhouse 1996a).

17. Both CGP and SJT have noticed a markedly more positive attitude toward suicide on the part of interns.

18. Note that we always have to allow for a tiny number of criminal acts of killing done in hospitals by clinicians because of twisted personal convictions.

19. Hendin 1996.

20. Rosenberg 1996.

21. Rosenberg 1996.

22. This may take the form of good advice given to patients who are psychologically unprepared to appreciate and act on it. It may also take the form of insensitively candid presentations of prognoses to patients.

23. This is a mixed bag of factors ranging from scarcity of resources to the psychological condition of a patient beset by great discomfort and anxiety.

24. Inadequate disclosure of treatment decisions is more elusive. For example, an elderly patient may contract pneumonia, which is not treated with antibiotics. But the patient may not be told clearly enough, or perhaps simply not told, that nothing is being done to counter the pneumonia. The pneumonia then may become a consideration in a suicidal decision in two different ways: It simply may preclude the point of such deliberation or it may figure in the deliberation as the decisive negative factor on the side of choosing self-destruction. Either way, the potential suicidist's autonomy is contravened. The counterpoint here is an extremely difficult question that shades off into epistemology, namely, the degree of capacity for autonomous decision-making by someone who is under tremendous pressure due to a pathological condition.

25. This doesn't refer to patients who are clinically depressed, but simply to those feeling the effects of appalling prognoses.

26. From various conversations one of us has had about this point, it seems that the primary fear people have is *loss of control* over their situations when hospitalized. There were many references to reassuring and often condescending generalities offered by attending clinicians in answer to questions about treatment and prognoses. The feeling that one isn't being told enough breeds concern that things may be done without one's authorization or even knowledge. It's especially true of the elderly that they fear that clinicians tend to treat them paternalistically.

27. It's also the case that patients are almost always strangers to attending clinicians, so the idea of malice toward them is seen as even more bizarre.

28. Including, of course, not treating someone beyond providing sedation.

29. See Anders 1997; see also Coutts 1997.

30. We're not using the term in its pejorative sense, but simply in its original sense of something done for pay.

31. CGP thinks that it's possible that aging baby boomers have only served as

a catalyst for a long overdue change in attitude toward technological maintenance of biologically unviable life. However, it is more likely that other and significantly deeper factors are at work. One of these could be growing generational resentment prompted by ever-increasing taxation not compensated for by greater opportunity. In most informal discussions CGP has had with colleagues in their thirties and early forties, the view was consistently expressed that older people's expectations are too high and that they ought to make way for younger people who expect considerably less from life. This was often put in terms of economic factors, but it took little pressing to bring up health-resources concerns. In this connection, it must be remembered that the somewhat extended life spans enjoyed since roughly the 1930s are a historically recent phenomenon and may not be permanent.

32. Of course, such consultation yields only the judgment confirmation of peers. Adherents of the slippery slope argument quickly point out that consultative decisions about assisted suicide will be foregone conclusions if clinicians are trained to consider assisted suicide as a readily available way of dealing with hard cases.

33. Some will not accept these pressures as extraneous, arguing that the cost of health care is an intrinsic element in prognosis and treatment.

34. Note that we are not considering here cases in which someone is comatose or in such agony that they are unable to form or express a desire to continue to live.

35. In the Latimer case in Canada, for example, someone enduring great suffering but unable to communicate or perhaps even form the desire to die was assumed by her parents to want to die.

36. It isn't at all clear that we'll continue to respect individuals as the final arbiters regarding their own lives. Rosenberg points out that although advocates of assisted suicide presently "invoke the empowerment of the patient, it is the clinician who is, in fact, effectively empowered" (Rosenberg 1996). He and Hendin intend this as a telling point against legalizing assisted suicide, but it may be no more than a statement of societal fact. Perhaps we can no longer afford to leave it to individuals whether they will live or die if their choosing to live puts unacceptable burdens on us. Society soon may be prepared to systematically withdraw or not initiate treatment when the cost and effort are too high relative to the care of others. In effect, that would be to turn the clock back to a time when life-sustaining treatment wasn't available to anyone, regardless of resources. It is sobering to remember that high-tech life-sustaining treatment isn't available now to the larger part of the planet's population.

37. What we're seeing in the development of managed health-care is continuing clashes between broad communal standards and professional standards regarding provision of costly treatment. See Anders 1997.

38. It is extremely important to note that such indecision or ambivalence need not be mere vacillation; irresolution may be prompted by difficulties in reconciling moral or religious values and the desire to die.

39. But see Hendin 1996 and Rosenberg 1996.

40. The Dutch situation is complex. Unlike Australia's Northern Territory case, assisted suicide isn't legal as such, nor is it specifically illegal. Rather, assisted suicide is not prosecuted as homicide or as abetting homicide except in cases when there is cause to do so.

41. Australia's Northern Territories assisted suicide and voluntary euthanasia legislation went into effect in July 1996 and was struck down on March 25, 1997. However, the vote was quite close: thirty-eight to thirty-three. Four people availed themselves of the law while it was in force. See "Australia Strikes Down a State Suicide Law," *New York Times*, March 25, 1997.

42. Here we again need to exclude clinical ethicists.

43. Pear 1997.

44. Kolata 1996b, 1997c.

45. Caplan interview, *Frontline*, 1996. Caplan isn't opposed to assisted suicide in principle; what he opposes is its likely abuse in a time of diminishing resources and an overtaxed health-care system:

> [U]ntil . . . I'm convinced that assisted suicide is the . . . option of last resort in the way that I think many of its proponents hope and wish it to be, until I see that societal commitment, I'm going to stand against it. . . . It's not that I think I can't be given cases individually where I would say yes. . . . I've been present—I haven't done it, but I've been present—at some assisted suicides, so I can hardly say that my ethics lead me to absolute opposition in believing that it is immoral.

46. Pear 1997.

47. In the main, the reference here includes clinical ethicists.

48. Nor is the eclipsing of value interests the only risk. Distinctions are increasingly being drawn among prudential interests. One of us thinks that an example of this is the way early-diagnosis Alzheimer's patients, who still have a significant prudential interest in survival, may "get written off very very quickly" by clinicians "who decide that their other illnesses are not worth treating" (Kolata 1997a). The other of us disagrees, not having witnessed such writing off of patients purely on the basis of being diagnosed with Alzheimer's disease.

49. It has emerged that prudential interests pose much less of a problem. In fact, we've seen that it's the relatively straightforward assessment of prudential interests that raises difficulties with reasoning, motives, and value interests.

50. This is a difficult case. Clinical ethicists may well side more with clinicians here than with theoreticians.

51. By this we mean the basic and usually unexamined assumptions operant in theoreticians' and clinicians' perceptions of the issue of assisted suicide. Another way of putting this point is to say that the differences between theoreticians and clinicians have to do with how much trouble each group looks for in assessing the permissibility of suicide.

52. Battin 1984:304. Note that Battin is speaking about depressed indi-

viduals, but the points made apply even more to individuals needing to decide whether they should live or die.

53. Battin 1984:304.

54. Rosenberg 1997.

55. It should be noted that flawless reasoning and motivation do not suffice, by themselves, for medically assisted suicide if neither the individual's condition nor the prognosis warrants self-destruction. A person could have good reasons to commit suicide because their values and priorities override their interest in survival, but if that person is in good health, there is no question of assisted suicide being provided in a medical context. We are nowhere near a point when a healthy individual can walk into a hospital and be given assistance in the commission of suicide because they want to, say, protest a government policy or because they fear exposure as a criminal.

56. There is a parallel here with abortion. However deplorable the more extreme tactics of those opposed to abortion, there can be no question that their persistent opposition serves as a check on the practice. For one thing, clinicians and institutions are circumspect about conducting the practice; for another, the arguments against abortion are kept prominently before the public and thus before individuals contemplating abortion.

57. This is another difficult case. On the whole, clinical ethicists are probably best counted as theoreticians here.

58. It bears reiterating that prudential interests are also defined by professional standards and may themselves differ significantly from prudential interests as perceived by the wider community.

7

A RECAPITULATION

In this chapter we recapitulate the major points discussed in earlier ones. Our aim is not only to reiterate key ideas but also to amplify a little and shift emphases slightly in order to further clarify what we've said.

Assisted suicide is practiced now in the form of cessation of treatment and some more intrusive methods.[1] Our contention is that assisted suicide soon will be socially accepted and more widely available to some patients, whether or not it is formally legalized. It is an idea whose time has come, despite many questions and problems. But questions of greater acceptance and legality aside, since assisted suicide *is* practiced, we immediately need consistent ethical guidance to govern it. Despite extensive efforts to provide guidance, there's little consistency in the principles used to test for and justify the permissibility of assisting suicide. Moral, religious, and professional priorities vary, and patients considering self-destruction may find themselves in institutional contexts that make getting help impossible or, alternatively, too easy. However, more serious than inconsistency is an ultimately vitiating divergence of ethical theory and clinical practice. The fundamental reason for the divergence is that trying to meet theoretical requirements as well as practical demands in dealing with assisted suicide generates irresolvable conflicts. Compromise is the only way out of these day-to-day impasses, so we need to achieve a balance of theoretical and practical considerations in decisions about the permissibility of assisted suicide.

Achieving such a balance calls for the legalization or at least the social condoning of the practice. Ensuring that the requisite balance is achieved will prove extremely difficult, if not impossible,[2] if assisted suicide continues to be practiced surreptitiously or to be misdescribed to gain its acceptance in particular cases. But even more important is the social acceptance of assisted suicide, which would enable its eventual legalization. The main obstacles to social acceptance are the view that suicide is irrational and the claim that sanctioning assisted suicide is stepping onto a slippery slope leading inexorably to expedient murder.

We've attempted to dispel the view that suicide is irrational or pathological by offering criteria that show when suicide is a rational option for an individual—that is, when the choice of suicide is unimpaired, is soundly motivated, and best serves a person's interests. When suicide satisfies these conditions, it is permissible to assist its commission. As for the slippery slope argument, it claims that legalized assisted suicide would turn compassionate aid in dying to expedient elimination of those who are terminally ill, severely disabled, or simply too old. We contend that despite appearances, the argument isn't a factual or empirical one but is about the cumulative effects of fostering new attitudes toward life and health care. We think that the possible slide has to do with how clinicians' assessments of patients' interests are rooted in the standards of a professional community, and how those standards may differ significantly from those of society at large. Our suggestion, then, is that rather than seeing the slippery slope argument as a possibly preclusive maneuver, we should see it as a valid and worthwhile caveat.

Within the structure provided by our criteria and reconstrual of the slippery slope argument, the details of the previous chapters mainly had to do with how theoretical requirements for assisted suicide may be eroded in application to actual cases, and how assisted suicide may slip into being something different: either unduly influenced self-destruction or voluntary euthanasia. The point is not that influenced self-destruction or voluntary euthanasia is necessarily unwarranted, only that weakening of the theoretical requirements—that suicidal deliberation be unimpaired, that suicidal motivation be cogent, and that suicide best serve an individual's interests—may result in an act no longer being *suicide*, in which case different ethical,[3] moral, and legal requirements would apply.

THE NATURE OF THEORY-PRACTICE CONFLICTS

As we've noted, the key to understanding the conflict of theory and practice, with respect to the permissibility of assisted suicide, is that the
requirements of the theoretical and the demands of the practical are
often irreconcilable. The simplest but the most important reason for conflict is that theory is inherently general, whereas practice is irreversibly
specific and contextual. This is why it appears that in trying to establish
rational and ethical guidelines for the permissibility of suicide, theoreticians "try to apply logic to a situation that defies it."[4] There are probably
few human psychological and behavioral situations so thoroughly
defined by personal and particular considerations as suicide. The factors
relevant to consideration of self-destruction are so peculiar to individuals and particular circumstances that they seem to defy effective generalization, if not logic itself. Clinicians who care for the dying appreciate this point all too well, so they tend to resist "theory." But their
resistance isn't really to theory as such; their resistance is to theory's
intrinsic generality, and hence its apparent irrelevance to the particular
cases with which they deal. Yet we can't afford *not* to provide theoretical
guidelines for the permissibility of assisted suicide. That would be to
risk allowing practices to become established that would vary unacceptably according to individual perceptions, emotional responses, and
values, as well as according to institutional policies and constraints, and
even according to regional economic realities.

Some argue that the logic governing individuals' decisions in specific
circumstances about whether to take their lives "cannot be transferred to
any other person or time."[5] But even if society must allow individuals to
work out their own logic about their own deaths, it can't risk leaving it to
individuals to decide on their own whether to help someone *else* to die.
This is especially true of clinicians, who are entrusted—and licensed—
to care for the patients in their charge. However hard to achieve, there
must be guidance and accountability if someone participates in another's
self-destruction.[6] We really have no choice. The mistake, though, is to
think that we can develop regulations that will be effective in governing
all cases of assisted suicide. The particulars of individual cases will
always require adjustment of applicable principles. Our only recourse is
to strive for a reasonable balance of theoretical and practical considerations in decisions about whether or not to provide assistance in suicide.
We need guidelines and standards that incorporate enough theory to

establish and maintain the requisite measure of uniformity in what is and isn't allowable but allow adequate leeway for contextual fine-tuning and don't paralyze people by demanding rigid conformity. At least as important, we need to train clinicians to be sensitive to the need to balance the requirements of theory and the demands of practice.

To enable compromise between the opposing pulls of theoretical prerequisites and practical necessities, the first thing that needs to be done is to show that suicide can be rational in the sense of being the best thing to do in a given situation. This is also required to enable assistance in its commission. Otherwise, assisting commission of suicide would be to enable an irrational self-destructive act, and so would be compounding a wrong. The job of our criteria is to show that suicide can be rational and so may be assisted when it can't be committed without help.[7] The criteria state the minimal and most general theoretical requirements for rational suicide and thus for permissible assistance in the commission of suicide.

Recall that our criteria for rational suicide determine that an autonomous act of self-killing is an instance of rational suicide when (1) suicide is a genuine option for the agent, chosen after deliberation consistent with accepted standards of reasoning and unimpaired by error, false beliefs, or lack of relevant information; and (2) the agent's motivating values are cogent to others, not unduly contravening the agent's interests; and (3) suicide is in the agent's interests, not causing more harm than continuing to live. Having discussed them in some detail, we can now condense the criteria by saying that to be rational, suicide must be an autonomous choice that is unimpaired, is done for cogent reasons, and best serves the agent's interests.

Interpretation of the criteria raises difficult issues, but in light of the need to better integrate theory and practice, some of those questions gain priority over others that, though equally important, are less pressing in the present context. The key question we were left with in considering the first criterion's application in medical contexts had to do with whether the proper focus of assessment for possible impairment is an individual's particular reasoning or overall competence. That is, the question is whether clinicians should evaluate a patient's suicidal deliberation in detail, or whether it's enough for them to evaluate that patient's general ability to make major treatment decisions. The former requirement seems to put an impossible burden on clinicians; the latter may jeopardize the rationality of patients' suicidal choices, which is the warrant for provision of assistance in suicide.

The question we were left with regarding the second criterion had to do with the significance of patients' suicidal motives relative to hopeless prognoses. Acceptable motivation for choosing to relinquish life is a requirement for rational suicide, but in medical contexts, suffering and bleak prognoses seem to relegate motives to a secondary status. As suffering escalates and prospects wane, it seems to make less and less difference why a patient wants to relinquish life. What seems to matter most at that point is that the patient does want to escape an intolerable situation. In a sense, clinicians' understanding of patients' conditions and likely futures seems to displace patients' own reasons for choosing not to live. But the danger theoreticians—and legislators—worry about is that the relative unimportance of motives will be too readily assumed, leading to irrational motives being increasingly ignored as accession to requests for assisted suicide becomes routine.

The question raised by the third criterion appears similar to the one posed by the second, because it seems that the need to protect patients' value interests also decreases in those cases in which the importance of motives diminishes, i.e., when prudential interests become minimal or negative. However, the questions are only superficially similar. What emerged in chapter 5 is that value interests may run counter to assessments of prudential interests, even when patients have requested assistance in suicide. What is at issue is autonomy, so value interests must be decisive. Regardless of how clear it is to clinicians that patients' prudential interests in survival are minimal or negative, patients' value interests take precedence with respect to the commission of suicide and its timing. Someone may want to die, may understand that death is in their best interests, may request aid in dying, and still delay suicide because of difficulty reconciling it with moral or religious views. Or patients' preparedness to die simply may not be in line with clinicians' expectations about timing.

In the case of the second criterion and motivation, the issue isn't opposition between patients and clinicians about suicide but the adequacy of patients' motives. In those cases, patients' value interests coincide with clinicians' assessments of their prudential interests, so the only question is whether the latter assessments suffice to ignore patients' problematic reasons. The question posed by the third criterion is how to determine when prudential interests are minimal or negative enough to allow clinicians to take requests for assistance in suicide at face value and not pursue value interests. The question is also about the propriety of exerting warranted influence on irresolute patients.[8] In effect, the question is less about when to assist suicide than it is about when a case of potential assisted suicide slides into being one of voluntary euthanasia.

All three of these questions have to do with relating third-party assessments of an individual's circumstances to that individual's own perceptions and judgments. In the cases that concern us, the third parties in question are clinicians, either working in medical institutions or providing home care. Clinicians have knowledge and experience that not only enable them to make expert assessments of patients' circumstances but also dispose them to perceive patients' circumstances differently enough to occasion serious conflicts with patients' assessments of their own circumstances. And to special knowledge and experience, we have to add clinicians' values, the effects of their particular working environments, their age,[9] a measure of inurement to death and dying, varying interpretations of professional and institutional policies, and individual professional and personal priorities. There is also the inescapable fact that patients sick enough to be considering suicide will be at their most vulnerable, and so easily influenced by those on whom they are dependent. There's a real danger, then, of hidden contravention[10] of patient autonomy by such things as undue influencing of suicidal deliberation, indifference to ambivalence, and compromising treatment decisions inadequately conveyed to patients.[11]

In line with our more concise restatement of the criteria for rational suicide, we can also restate the questions about the criteria more briefly: First, in evaluating the permissibility of assisted suicide, should assessment focus on suicidal deliberation or on general competence? Second, when does patient motivation become immaterial to decisions about providing assisted suicide? And third, when should patients' value interests cease to be decisive against clinicians' negative assessments of patients' prudential interests in survival? But note that since we are dealing with assisted suicide, the point of the second and third questions primarily has to do with when clinicians may take a request for assistance in commission of suicide at face value and not pursue the soundness of patients' motives or the precise nature of their value interests. The point isn't about when clinicians can perform euthanasia; the questions aren't about when clinicians can make decisions on behalf of patients.[12]

These three questions in effect mark out a continuum running from fully autonomous self-destruction to acceptance of death at someone else's hands. In other words, different answers to these questions take us from full-fledged suicide through influenced suicide[13] to voluntary euthanasia.[14] In medical contexts, the incremental points on the continuum are set by decreasing capacity for autonomous action on the part of patients and/or increasing involvement by clinicians in patients' deliberations and decisions. What determines how different the answers are to questions about focus of assessment, motivation, and interests are patients' medical conditions and prospects. Generally, the worse the conditions and prospects, the more warranted the participation of clinicians in patients' choices. That is, the worse off the patients are, and the bleaker their prospects, the more clinicians can discount patients' reasoning, motives, and value interests and base their own decisions and actions on their expert assessment of patients' prudential interests.

The worries we've discussed regarding application of our three criteria come to this: How can we ensure that clinicians will participate in patients' choices in a warranted manner that doesn't erode patients' autonomy or the rationality of their suicidal decisions? As we've stressed, the main concern here *isn't* that clinicians will behave in ways prompted by hidden agendas or malice. The worry is that their training, experience, and compassion may unduly color their perceptions and prompt them to involve themselves too effectively in patients' suicidal decisions.[15]

When we translate the foregoing questions into social-policy terms, the worry about clinicians having too much influence on patients' suicidal choices becomes the question of whether social and professional acceptance of assisted suicide would establish policies that may eventually dispossess too many patients of the final say over relinquishing their lives.[16] If policies ensue that contravene patients' autonomy, we may well begin a slide down a slippery slope.

Consider that at present a patient in a coma may be removed from a life-support system on the basis of the family's request and satisfaction of applicable institutional and legal conditions.[17] We can imagine that under tough new policies and laws, some conscious and competent patients might be put in the same category as comatose patients, on the strength of hopeless prognoses and excessively costly life support.[18] The point would be to enable termination of life support and to remove the need to treat certain conditions such as pneumonia contracted while hospitalized.[19] Family or surrogates' consent and attending physicians' decisions might be deemed adequate regardless of the patients' wishes. The obvious parallel is to how someone may be committed for psychiatric examination, or even more permanently, quite against their will.

At present, one condition for cessation of treatment of incompetent or comatose patients is that in the absence of patient consent, there must be a "substituted" decision, i.e., an appropriate individual must make a decision based on what the patient would most likely want or would request if able to do so. This requires some knowledge of the patient and close attention to whether the patient ever said anything applicable to the situation, such as that they wouldn't want to live under certain conditions. There may be documentary evidence of patient wishes, such as a living will or advanced directive.[20] When a substituted decision is unavailable for some reason—e.g., the patient has no close relatives or friends—another condition requires that a surrogate make a decision that is deemed to be in the patient's best interests. The appeal is to the interests a society considers to be basic. But those interests may be reconceived and are never assessed in a vacuum. In a given society, individuals' basic interests may be redefined because they are always circumscribed by the effects that satisfying those interests has on the interests of others. We can imagine a hard-pressed society, forced by scarce resources and increasing numbers, to say to its hopeless medical cases: We can't care for you, but we can't just abandon you, so we'll help you to die.[21] Though this sounds brutal to us now, many would argue that it's morally *less* repugnant to give someone a dignified, peaceful death than to keep them in facilities offering minimal or inadequate care or to dump them on their families. A society might begin to withdraw life support of various sorts from patients who are still competent to reject assisted suicide or voluntary euthanasia. We must remember that, in the end, what causes death in such cases is the underlying condition, that life support is only a delaying tactic, and that society can decide that such support is a conditional privilege rather than a right.

SHARPENING THE FOCUS

So far, we have the theoretical requirements that suicide and assisted suicide be unimpaired, cogently motivated, and for the best. Applying these requirements in evaluating cases of assisted suicide in medical contexts prompts us to ask whether impairment has to do with suicidal deliberation or general competence, whether motivation becomes immaterial at some deteriorative point, and when expert assessment of patients' prudential interests suffices to permit inattention to their value interests. The picture we've tried to paint is of these theoretical requirements being not so much contravened as eroded by practical and contextual factors in their application. This isn't a process peculiar to assisted suicide in medical contexts. *Any* practice conducted by a number of people over a period of time involves some erosion of its principles in day-to-day application. The concern is to avoid *systemic* erosion. The main source of possible systemic erosion in the case of assisted suicide in medical contexts is disproportionate variance in professional and lay perceptions of the circumstances that occasion assisted suicide.[22]

Variance in clinicians' and patients' perceptions of their own circumstances, when assisted suicide has been requested or seems indicated, threatens patients' autonomy and the rationality of their suicides because of the pivotal fact that patients are precisely that: *patients*. They are disempowered by illness, and often by suffering and despondency. They are dependent on professionals who have a great deal of both obvious and subtle control over their treatment and options. But the threat posed hasn't much to do with clinicians willfully exercising their power or control. The reality, and our working assumption, is that clinicians are genuinely disposed to do what is best for their patients. The trouble lies in this very disposition. There may be inadvertent abuse of control caused by convictions about what's best for patients.[23] Clinicians may act in ways described in the literature as paternalistic or "parentalistic,"[24] which basically means that clinicians feel warranted in acting "as if they had the authority and concern of a parent."[25] Clinicians may feel what Hendin describes as the need "for closure and control when available technical tools are no longer relevant."[26] The result is that they may deliberately or inadvertently press patients to act before they're ready. This doesn't have to involve direct urging of patients; it may be much more subtle and be limited to no more than manner, tone of voice, and all the other little things we do to convey our views. Another possibility is that clinicians may influence patients who either haven't seriously considered suicide or have but are ambivalent. The influencing may also be deliberate or inadvertent, direct or indirect. In any case, patients' autonomy may be jeopardized or contravened by pressure or forceful suggestion, and the rationality of their suicides may be weakened to the extent that they're brought to choose suicide when they might not have done so if left to themselves.

There are, of course, times when clinicians are warranted in acting paternalistically in patients' best interests, particularly when patients' states of mind preclude them from making significant decisions or even complying with instructions important to their well-being. But in the case of assisted suicide, paternalism has no place.[27] Clinicians may feel certain that it's in a patient's interests to die in order to avoid unnecessary and intense suffering, and they may balk at what they see as counterproductive and intrusive probing of that patient's state of mind.[28] Clinicians' convictions will be even stronger when patients have requested assistance in suicide, but "[e]ven if the ends are the patient's own ends, to treat him as a means to them is to undermine his humanity insofar as humanity consists in choosing and being able to judge one's own ends."[29] Choosing one's own ends and, in the cases at issue, choosing one's own *end* and its timing are central to being an autonomous person. Autonomy tolerates no measure of paternalistic influencing or hastening of someone's self-destruction.[30]

The occasion for unwarranted paternalism regarding assisted suicide is generated by juxtaposition of patients' perceptions as conditioned by suffering, fear, and despondency and clinicians' perceptions as conditioned by training, experience, and confidence that they know what's best for those in their care. This juxtaposition can have varied results, but the most worrying is that patients may be unduly influenced and avail themselves of a "soothing moral shroud"[31] seemingly or actually offered by attending clinicians. It's just this sort of possibility that drives theoreticians' caution, and why they insist on strict application of the criteria for rational suicide.

The fundamental fact is that there's an irreducible difference between clinicians' and patients' perceptions of the same medical situations. Patients' perceptions of their own situations are strongly colored by the *uniqueness* of those situations in their experience. Clinicians' perceptions of patients' situations are as strongly colored by the *familiarity* of those situations in their own professional experience.

These divergent perspectives ensure that patients will be considerably more tentative and ambivalent about suicidal decisions than clinicians, especially about the timing of even the most fervently desired death. But this isn't just because it's their *own* deaths that are being considered. The point is that ordinary people, who find themselves considering suicide to avoid enduring what survival may bring, simply haven't faced that choice before. They won't have thought about it. They won't have a basis for comparison. They won't know how to assess their own prudential interests. They'll be hindered in their deliberation by their value interests, because they won't know how to realign their priorities.[32] Their motives for wanting to die will often be rationalizations that obscure more than they justify.[33] In short, even if unimpaired, most patients' reasoning about self-destruction likely won't be sound. Their motives will be muddled. They won't discern their own best interests effectively.

Contrary to the plight of patients, clinicians have been through it all before: They've dealt with cases in which suicide is the wisest course of action, and they've dealt with fearful and confused patients and families. Clinicians have extensive experience in assessing patients' prudential interests. They have recourse to detailed prognoses and expert peer support. They understand how intense suffering can make patients' value interests evaporate and effectively make patients' reasoning and motivation immaterial to their desire to cease to live as they are living. Experience can't help but have a tempering effect, so clinicians don't see death in the dramatic terms patients do.[34] This may incline some clinicians to be overly brisk in acceding to requests for assisted suicide, thereby intimidating patients. Patients who request assisted suicide in a moment of despair may feel locked into their "choice," and their autonomy is thereby eroded or contravened.[35]

What we have, then, is that even if there's agreement on the criteria for rational suicide, their application is far from straightforward because of inconsistency among assessments due to variance in perceptions. With respect to value interests in particular, what some reject as wretched and intolerable physical conditions, others find acceptable in light of moral or religious prohibition against self-destruction. In "the maelstrom that is the human psyche as death nears,"[36] any number of things affect perceptions and the weight given the many factors relevant to the deliberation of suicide. When we add the complexities attendant on *others* deciding whether or not to assist in suicide, it looks as if we can't impose regulative order on people deciding to relinquish their lives or to help others do so. It's quite possible that social and professional acceptance of assisted suicide would worsen perception difficulties. The variance of patients' and clinicians' perceptions could be made intractable by introducing the element of conventional availability of assisted suicide into an equation presently weighted in favor of caution and circumspection by prohibitions. Clinicians dealing with assisted suicide as a conventional treatment option would be even further removed from their patients' perspectives on self-destruction.

Regardless of its being practiced in the past and at present,[37] it's undeniable that the availability of socially and professionally—and perhaps legally—sanctioned assisted suicide would create a very different situation from the current one. At present, assisted suicide often must be disguised, and clinicians have to decide whether to defy the law in spirit, if not in detail, to comply with patients' requests for assistance in self-destruction. Certainly the number of cases of assisted suicide would increase if the practice were condoned, and especially if it were legalized. Clinicians who are willing to provide assistance in the commission of suicide but are restrained by the threat of criminal charges wouldn't have to worry about such charges. Others, ambivalent about the morality of assisting suicide, would find reassurance in social and professional acceptance of the practice. Medical training would also be significantly affected; clinicians trained in an atmosphere of tolerance regarding assisted suicide almost certainly would be considerably more prone to accede to patient requests for help in self-destruction.

The basic issue is about the consequences of facilitating actions that are presently hemmed by legal, moral, and cultural prohibitions. Unfortunately, we have little to go on with respect to divining how things will turn out if we sanction assisted suicide. Most theoreticians think that if prohibitions are removed, formally or informally, assisted suicide must be governed by punctilious adherence to standards established to determine permissibility. Clinicians and some clinical ethicists argue that what controls the practice of assisted suicide is in place *now* and won't be materially changed by broader acceptance or legalization. In their view, what controls the present practice of assisted suicide, and will continue to control legalized practice, is a combination of sound medical procedures, professional principles, and basic humanity.

THE DILEMMA: KNOWING ONE'S OWN
OR ANOTHER'S MIND

Most of what we've said so far, and a great deal of what others have said, ultimately has to do with how we can establish what a person caught in "the maelstrom"[38] of approaching death really wants to do. Not only is this question prior to the question of whether what they want to do is *moral*, it's even prior to the question of whether what they want to do is *rational*.[39] Our arguments and cautions about reasoning, motivation, and interests all center on first establishing what an individual actually intends. But clarity and resoluteness of intention are very elusive for most people when what is at issue is survival. It is this basic truth that generates all the problems and arguments about the oppositions of sound and impaired reasoning, clear and confused motives, and conflicts between value and prudential interests. Our recourse when faced with perplexity about intentions, whether in others or in ourselves, is *what is in character*. We rely on abiding values and priorities to resolve irresoluteness about many of our choices.

In an amicus curiae brief presented to the U. S. Supreme Court, six of North America's most noted moral philosophers addressed the various pros and cons of clinician-assisted suicide, providing a two-step argument justifying state involvement in what many consider to be a purely medical issue.[40] In his introduction to the published brief, Ronald Dworkin summarized the argument:

> First, [the argument] defines a very general moral and constitutional principle—that every competent person has the right to make momentous personal decisions which invoke fundamental religious or philosophical convictions about life's value for himself. Second, it recognizes that people may make such momentous decisions impulsively or out of emotional depression, when their act does not reflect their enduring convictions.[41]

People's "enduring convictions" offer the most reliable standard with respect to whether or not something they request, such as assistance in suicide, reflects a sound decision[42] on their part or only an expression of despair or desperation.[43] Because people sometimes *do* make serious decisions for various reasons that don't reflect their "enduring convictions," the brief stresses that "in some circumstances a state has the constitutional power to override" the right to decide to relinquish life "to protect citizens from mistaken but irrevocable acts of self-destruction." The application of the argument to the issue of assisted suicide turns on how "[s]tates may be allowed to prevent assisted suicide by people who—it is plausible to think—would later be grateful if they were prevented from dying."[44]

We are in general agreement with the brief's argument, but there is a problem that is key to the acceptance of the practice of assisted suicide in medical contexts. The argument essentially grants people the right to choose to relinquish life for reasons of deep conviction. Philosophical convictions clearly include valuing life only so long as it is judged worth living and considering it best forfeited when value and prudential interests in survival turn minimal or negative. The argument's second step acknowledges that people may choose to forfeit life "impulsively or out of emotional depression," to which we would add "or because of undue influence." So far, the brief's argument is entirely in accord with what we maintain. The trouble arises with determining that a patient requesting assisted suicide might "later be grateful if . . . prevented from dying." It would appear that the only basis for that judgment would be *positive assessment of prudential interests*. The assumption is that clinicians and family members shouldn't comply with requests for suicide made by patients judged to have a significant prudential interest in survival. This is precisely the sort of situation our second criterion guards against: the dismissal of patients' value interests in light of assessment of their prudential interests. There's also a worrying implication: If prudential interests suffice to override value interests in *preventing* compliance with requests for assisted suicide, then it seems to follow that minimal or negative prudential interests suffice to *accede* to such requests without further probing of value interests. This is just the concern we explore in chapter 5, that value interests may be unjustifiably diminished in importance and people may be unduly influenced or hurried in commission of suicide.

There's no question in our minds that the brief's conclusion is correct that "[e]ach individual has a right to make the 'most intimate and personal choices central to personal dignity and autonomy.' " It is also certainly correct that "[t]hat right encompasses the right to exercise some control over the time and manner of one's death."[45] However, though it's of great importance that the courts resolve the rights issue, it's still more important that the ongoing practice of assisted suicide in medical contexts[46] be conducted in ways that ensure that when patients request assistance in suicide and are granted that assistance, they commit suicide in accordance with their "enduring convictions." It goes without saying that it's as important that the future practice of assisted suicide, whether or not legalized, be equally well governed. As we've seen, the real problems are in the interpretation and application of the criteria for rational suicide and the permissibility of assisted suicide. To ensure that suicide and assisted suicide are in accordance with enduring convictions,[47] some order must be imposed on the emotional and interactional turmoil generated by someone choosing whether or not to forfeit life and others deciding whether or not to help. Proper assessment of reasoning, motivation, and interests is necessary to determine whether an individual's self-destructive choice is in line with who they have been during their lifetime and isn't just a result of who they've briefly become while experiencing great stress, suffering, and vulnerability to undue influences.

The picture usually painted by advocates of assisted suicide is one of fully competent people coolly assessing their options and making sound choices with the support of attending clinicians and loved ones. In this picture, the suicidist's autonomy is never in question. Others' involvement in the decision and act is supportive, not intrusive. But cases like that are very rare. The reality is that choosing to relinquish life in the face of great suffering or a prolonged death is seldom a clear-cut decision, and even more rarely is there a solid consensus among members of Hendin's dynamic interactional system comprising patient, clinicians, family, and close friends.[48] Far more likely are scenarios in which patients want to relinquish life, clinicians think that self-destruction is unwarranted, and family members, to the extent that they're involved,[49] are divided; or in which clinicians see suicide as best serving patients' interests, patients vacillate, and family members are again divided. These diverse scenarios are complicated by institutional policies and further complicated—sometimes acutely—by the influence that the involved parties have on one another. Patients may be influenced in one way by clinicians' desire for closure and in a contrary way by their families' misgivings or disapproval; clinicians may be influenced in one direction by families' entreaties and in a contrary direction by patients' desperation; families may be influenced in a positive fashion by clinicians' expert judgments and in a negative fashion by patients' ambivalence or confusion. In fact, the very diversity of interplaying views, and their emotional nature, may dispose patients to make rash decisions because of anxiety over the turmoil they are causing.

This diversity seems to make it impossible to effectively apply theoretically devised criteria for rational suicide. Applying the criteria for rational suicide under such variable and emotional conditions looks like "try[ing] to apply logic to a situation that defies it."[50] But without application of the criteria, patients may make disastrously impulsive, confused, or unduly influenced requests and decisions. Additionally, clinicians could rely only on their own judgments and possibly inconsistent responses to particular circumstances. And perhaps most dangerous, institutional policies could be too heavily instrumental in determining outcomes. Even if practical clinical situations involving assisted suicide appear to defy "logic" or theoretical systemization, that doesn't mean that we should—or that we *can*—throw up our hands and simply count on the goodwill and good sense of the parties involved. There must be genuine, serious efforts at imposing rational governance and uniformity on how decisions about assisted suicide are made by clinicians charged with the well-being of patients.[51] Hendin may be right that we can't properly monitor, much less control, how people come to choose to forfeit their lives. But we *must* monitor and control how *others* participate in people's suicides, especially when those others are licensed to care for patients they may help to die.

The apparent defiance of "logic" brings us back to the difference between conceiving of the criteria for rational suicide as *prior* to and determinative of the permissibility of assisted suicide and conceiving of them as *derivative* from proven practice. Depending on the conception, we are best advised to rely either on preconditions or on what has been established as most productive and acceptable. Relying on preconditions leaves us plagued by problems with interpretation and application

of the criteria; but construing the criteria as following on accepted practice leaves us haunted by the possibility of anomalous or misconceived
practical elements gaining unwarranted acceptance. The dilemma comes
down to a question of trust. On the one hand, we can put our trust in
abstract universal principles to define and govern provision of assisted
suicide. The reasoning is that regulating principles must be *external* to
properly govern practice, and that accepted practice may contain elements that either erode patient autonomy or could too easily come to do
so if assisted suicide became a conventional treatment option. On the
other hand, we can put our trust in established practice judged to best
meet our needs and protect our interests over the long run. The reasoning
here is that the most efficacious and reliable regulating principles are
internal to practice, that practice is self-correcting, and that autonomy-
eroding elements will be discerned and compensated for over time.

There are two illuminating parallels we can draw at this point: a
legal one and an economic one. The legal parallel is with British
common law's reliance on precedents. The trust is that legislation is
honed over time and thus is fairer and more effective than slavish adherence to abstractly formulated laws. The economic parallel is with our
market economy's reliance on competition, supply, and demand to control prices and safeguard interests. The trust is that practices honed by
market forces and experience will better and more fairly regulate com-
merce than the imposition of strict rules. In both cases, tradition and
broad communal participation are deemed to be better regulators than
codification. One can take this confidence as well-grounded, and as
applicable to the assisted suicide issue, and argue that experience with
actual cases shows that confidence is warranted regarding the rationality
and humane nature of the present and foreseeable provision of assistance in suicide in medical contexts. Or one can take the confidence as
misplaced and argue that past and present practices are largely irrelevant to the issue of how assisted suicide will be dealt with once it
becomes conventional in the sense of becoming a socially and professionally accepted option—whether or not formally legalized.[52]

The parallels with legal and economic models suggest that the
choice between relying on abstractly formulated criteria for rational suicide and permissible assisted suicide or on practice-derived guidelines
is a false one. Despite the precedent and market-forces models, our legal
and economic systems combine both reliance on abstractly formulated
rules and practical adjustment of those rules. If assisted suicide gains
social and professional acceptance, it will certainly involve both abstract
criteria and rules and contextual interpretation of them. That goes

without saying. Our concern is with *priorities*. As we said in chapter 1, the pivotal issue generated by the conflicting requirements and demands of ethical theory and clinical practice is about whether abstract principles or what we called "the messy contours" of particular cases are given priority in making decisions about providing assistance in suicide. In arguing for balance between theory and practice, we intend to facilitate a duality in the practice of assisted suicide comparable to those dualities inherent in our legal and economic systems. But we remain divided on the question of whether theoretical or practical factors must be decisive in the hard judgments that need to be made when patients request help in relinquishing their lives.

What seems quite clear is that *training* may be the most crucial determinant of the rational and ethical practice of assisted suicide. Whether the appeal is to abstract principles or established practice, what is most important is how individual clinicians approach cases in which suicide becomes an issue. Whatever may be decided about the priority of the theoretical or the practical, medical training must be enriched with enough ethical content to ensure that medical practice continues to be sound once assisted suicide is more broadly accepted and possibly legalized. This means inculcating a sensitivity to, and an appreciation of, ethical-theoretical considerations. Training must also inculcate a certain measure of sociopolitical acumen. Clinicians must be able to recognize the different influences on them and to reflect effectively on their own interpretive predispositions. Additionally, there must be progress in understanding the exigencies of terminal illness, advanced age, and severe disability. If assisted suicide is socially and professionally accepted, and possibly widely legalized, it must be in order to deal with these exigencies, and not to provide a Draconian solution to the social and economic burdens they represent.[53]

NOTES

1. For example, recourse to large amounts of sedation when patients' pain justifies the dosages despite the high probability that they'll prove fatal.

2. A prerequisite for clinicians' properly understanding the need for balance, and how to achieve it, is *training*, and clinicians can't be trained in procedures banned by law.

3. Recall that *ethical* is being used to refer to professional codes.

4. Nuland 1997. Nuland adds: "If there is logic to be snatched from the maelstrom that is the human psyche as death nears, it is more likely to be found by the individuals living through each particular situation than by legislators, advocacy groups or the courts."

5. Nuland 1997. Nuland's claim is that "when a logical decision somehow arises out of the chaos surrounding death it is a very individual logic—that of the patient, family members and doctors, who are all struggling under the specific circumstances."

6. This works both ways; there must also be accountability and guidance regarding intervention in attempted suicide.

7. Again, it is necessary to be careful here. In some cases of assisted suicide, even though they are largely incapacitated, patients can perform the required action that directly causes death: e.g., taking pills provided or pushing a button, as in Dr. Kevorkian's machine. When patients are immobile, voluntary euthanasia must be performed. There is also a *practical* consideration. Most people can commit suicide in one way or another: e.g., stop eating or jump out a window. Many clinicians feel that since this is usually true, there isn't any need for them to be involved in patients' self-destruction. But patients shouldn't have to take their lives in ways that cause them unnecessary suffering. It isn't good enough to say to a bedridden patient: Fine, if you want to die, stop eating. If the means are available to help people to die with little or no pain, and quickly, it is to fail in one's obligations to patients to force them either to live in agony, because they lack the capacity to commit suicide by the means available to them, or to kill themselves in some way that causes them great suffering.

8. This is, of course, the hardest call: not only *when* something can be done, but also *what* is to be done. Whereas some patients find their conditions intolerable and have no value interest and possibly no prudential interest in survival, other patients in the same condition may desperately want to live out whatever time is left them—and this may be quite aside from what they *say* about suicide—or, more likely, may be irresolute. Their value interests aren't overridden by perceived loss of prudential interests in survival, as confused motives may be. The question then is what clinicians properly can do. Clearly, some sort of influence is in order, but it must be done in such a way as to protect the patient's autonomy, and not in a manner that takes undue advantage of the patient's vulnerability. Each case will be different and will call for great sensitivity to the particular patient's situation. This is Nuland's (1997) point about the particular "logic" of individuals in specific circumstances.

9. It is crucial to keep in mind that for patients, life is measured in weeks or months, whereas for attending clinicians, it is measured in decades. But at least as important are generational differences in how maintenance of tenuous life is viewed.

10. Such contravention will most likely be inadvertent; there is no suggestion intended that clinicians deliberately contravene patient autonomy.

11. See Krynski, Tymchuk, and Ouslander 1994.

12. As suggested, some influencing of irresolute patients may be in order, such as stressing the seriousness of a prognosis. The point isn't to coerce patients into suicide but to help them make up their minds.

13. But not *coerced* self-killing.

14. Of course, certain answers to these questions may take us to nonvoluntary or even involuntary euthanasia, when patients are beyond even willful acquiescence to euthanasia. However, those sorts of cases are not our concern in the present context.

15. Of course, this worry raises the complementary concern that overregulation of assisted suicide will make clinicians involve themselves too ineffectively.

16. We aren't naive enough to think that patients presently always have the final say; the point is about acknowledgment.

17. This may involve acquiring legal permission.

18. Limiting elderly patients' appeals of treatment-access denials is a step in that direction. See Pear 1997.

19. See Kolata 1997a.

20. See Annas 1991; Fisher and Meslin 1990; Gamble, McDonald, and Lichstein 1991; Kolata 1997d; McCrary and Botkin 1989; Robertson 1991; Samuels 1996; Stelter, Elliot, and Bruno 1992; Walker et al. 1995.

21. One of us remembers reading a newspaper story that illustrated the unacceptability of the alternative. It was reported to the police in Paris that a homeless person was lying unconscious under a bridge. The person was taken to a hospital and found to be suffering from dehydration, starvation, and severe exposure. The individual was hospitalized for six weeks and managed a fair recovery. The hospital then released the person, *and the police returned the individual to the bridge*. We've not been able to track down the story, which was little more than a filler, but it was reported in 1994.

22. In the 1990s, the clearest example of society coming to grips with this sort of variance is attempts to deal with racist attitudes held by some members of the police. In looking at systemic racism in some police departments, we see, at its worst, the split between, on the one hand, tacit professional attitudes and, on the other, a profession's *avowed* values and the wider society's values. There's no suggestion, of course, that clinicians harbor attitudes or values as repugnant as some that have emerged in recent court cases. The point is that in any profession, attitudes develop that may be significantly at odds with a profession's principles and societal expectations.

23. There is a good deal of controversy on this matter. Though "the dominant view [is] that there is justification for . . . paternalistic intervention against a person's wishes only when the person lacks mental competence . . . voices have been raised claiming that mental competence does *not* set a proper limit to beneficent intervention . . . for a person's own good" (Checkland and Silberfeld 1996:121).

24. See, for instance, Benjamin and Curtis 1986; Childress 1979; and Dworkin 1972. The term *parentalism* was introduced for its gender-neutrality and enjoyed a brief vogue, but it seems to have fallen into disuse. See also Checkland and Silberfeld 1996.

25. Benjamin and Curtis 1986:53.

26. Quoted in Rosenberg 1996; see Hendin 1996.

27. This is not to say that showing the authority and concern of a parent may not be warranted in cases calling for some form of euthanasia.

28. Attempting to clarify patients' value interests or motives can be traumatic for patients who have come to their decisions with great difficulty and are just managing to keep reservations and ambivalences in check. In contrast, *not* probing value interests or motives may allow patients who are ambivalent or irresolute to take their lives against deeper convictions and intentions.

29. Fried 1974:101.

30. As has been suggested before, it may be that we need to rethink the matter of autonomy; it may be that we will find we need to qualify it. However, here we must proceed on the basis of precisely what Fried says, namely, that "humanity consists in choosing and being able to judge one's own ends" (Fried 1974:101). We would add only the Kantian point noted earlier, that autonomous choices are choices made in accordance with reason.

31. Kristol 1993.

32. Both of us can provide, as can any clinician, numerous instances of literally pathetic desires and intentions had by dying people that precluded serious thought of self-destruction but were quite impossible.

33. One of us had a case in which a man in a terminal but not punishing condition wanted to die to rejoin his long-dead wife.

34. In a conversation with a clinician, one of us was told that death simply doesn't have "the same sting" for those working with terminal patients on a daily basis as it does for individual patients and theoreticians—one might add legislators, too.

35. Note that it is arguable that in some cases, when deterioration is advanced and the prognosis is dismal, patient autonomy *should* be overridden to some extent regarding aid in dying, so long as the patient has expressed a desire to die. As we will see in the final chapter, one of us isn't willing to consider such cases assisted suicide and thinks that they should be acknowledged as voluntary euthanasia.

36. Nuland 1997.

37. See Stevens 1997 for an interesting discussion of how assisted suicide ceased to be a medical decision and became a legal one with the Karen Ann Quinlan case. Note, though, that Stevens accepts, as do many clinical ethicists and clinicians, that cases of cessation of treatment, which usually are more properly described as voluntary or nonvoluntary euthanasia, are cases of assisted suicide.

38. Nuland 1997.

39. This point is evident in that one reason for choosing not to do something is that it's either immoral or irrational.

40. See Dworkin et al. 1997 on the brief and Stevens 1997 on the involvement of the courts. See also Steinfels 1997a.

41. Dworkin et al. 1997:41.

42. It's quite true that there are times when someone's well-being depends on them choosing to do something that is quite out of character and out of line with what have been their "enduring convictions." For example, someone trying to escape a psychologically stultifying situation or relationship may need to break with the person they've been all their lives in order to achieve a measure of freedom. It's possible that someone previously bound by, say, religious convictions may need to shed their faith in choosing to relinquish life when it's in their deepest interests to do so. But although we acknowledge such cases, they seem not to be the common rule.

43. Recall the point made earlier that despondency can make people's cherished values suddenly seem empty and pointless. See Battin 1984:304.

44. Dworkin et al. 1997:41.

45. Dworkin et al. 1997:47.

46. Dworkin's introduction to the amicus curiae brief gives figures in line with those we've given:

> For example, in a recent study in the state of Washington, which guaranteed respondents anonymity, 26 percent of doctors surveyed said they had received explicit requests for help in dying, and had provided, overall, lethal prescriptions to 24 percent of patients requesting them. In other studies, 40 percent of Michigan oncologists surveyed reported that patients had initiated requests for death, 18 percent said they had participated in assisted suicide, and 4 percent in "active euthanasia"—injecting lethal drugs themselves. In San Francisco, 53 percent of the 1,995 responding physicians said they had granted an AIDS patient's request for suicide assistance at least once. These statistics approach the rates at which doctors help patients die in Holland, where suicide is in effect legal (Dworkin et al. 1997:41–42).

47. We take it that reference to "enduring convictions" includes that these are rational convictions, as the alternative is to allow suicide and assisted suicide in accordance with *ir*rational convictions, which is certainly not the sense of the brief's appeal.

48. Hendin 1996; Rosenberg 1996.

49. In cases of assisted suicide, the condition is that patients be competent, hence the involvement of family members would be limited to advising, not to the making of decisions.

50. Nuland 1997.

51. See Kuhse 1997.

52. The allusion is again to the Netherlands, where assisted suicide is in effect legal, in that it is not prosecuted when conducted under specific circumstances.

53. Note that because this chapter is itself a recapitulation, no summary is offered.

8

NEW DECISIONS

"More and more, we are going to die when someone makes the decision that we are going to die."[1] The point, made by Marshall Perron, author of Australia's short-lived Northern Territories legislation on assisted suicide, is that thanks to modern medical technology, it's becoming the norm for clinicians to decide death's timing. Perron exaggerates in claiming that we soon *"will be able to keep virtually everyone alive indefinitely,"*[2] but his basic point is well taken. "Natural causes" or underlying pathological conditions are no longer the conclusive determinants of death that they once were. Technology has enabled us to delay natural death. Even if the extension of life is only a matter of weeks or even days, the fact is that with the application of enough technology, people can be kept alive well after the time they would have died if untreated or even if treated with methods only two or three decades old.[3] This capacity ranges from extending the lives of diabetics with insulin treatment, through dialysis for those with kidney damage, to keeping someone in a vegetative state alive on life-support apparatus. The significance of this capacity is that clinicians, though they certainly haven't conquered death, have gained a measure of control over when it actually occurs. The obverse is that it's become necessary for clinicians' patients to sometimes intervene regarding the maintenance of their own lives. There are now *decisions* to be made regarding death's timing.

A complicating element is that it's assumed by many, both health-care professionals and members of the general public, that because clinicians have the capacity to do so, they should sustain life *as a matter of course*. The principles of beneficence and especially nonmaleficence are assumed to require that clinicians do all they can to keep their patients alive for as long as possible. New technology therefore is seen not as posing new questions about the wisdom of its implementation but simply as enabling clinicians' to do better what they *should* do. As was alluded to earlier, this assumption raises a pressing question about the new control over death's timing: Are we prolonging life, or only protracting death? As Elisabeth Kübler-Ross puts it, "[w]e have to ask ourselves whether medicine is to remain a humanitarian . . . profession or [become] a new but depersonalized science in the service of prolonging life rather than diminishing human suffering."[4] In some intuitively clear sense, in particular cases, deciding whether we're prolonging life or only prolonging the process of dying depends on the quality of the extra time won by the use of technology. But as we saw in considering the possible conflict of value and prudential interests, determining what is worthwhile life involves myriad personal and social factors and seems to defy generalization.

The assumption that all available technology should be used to maintain life has put tremendous pressure on medical-care resources. Aside from the high cost of the technology itself and of its application, its use to keep people alive generates the additional costs of caring for those whose lives are prolonged or whose dying is protracted. As a consequence, we may be moving toward an ominous depreciation of "life that is dependent." Now that we're approaching a world population in the tens of billions, and now that resources are growing scarcer, arduous and costly maintenance of wholly dependent lives is becoming ever more grudging. Increasingly negative attitudes toward maintaining dependent, problematic life[5] might be more benign if the issue were simply the cost of caring for the terminally ill, the elderly, and the severely disabled in the sense of tending them and seeing to their basic needs.[6] That is, if individuals in these categories were living longer because of better lifelong nutrition and health care and therefore dying later and more slowly, then society would likely be more willing to bear the costs of their dying. But many, if not most, of these individuals are clinging to life longer, even though moribund, not because of stronger, more resistant constitutions but because their dying is being technologically protracted.

The assumption that all available means should be used to sustain life also makes it necessary—and often difficult—to justify *not* sustaining life for compassionate reasons. At present, not sustaining life when doing so becomes counterproductive is largely a matter of withholding or withdrawing treatment or not treating a pathological condition "aggressively." Less aggressive treatment doesn't always involve decisive measures such as not intubating patients or taking them off ventilators. It may be a matter of ceasing the use of antibiotics.[7] But what's important here aren't the details of how nature is allowed to take its course. What's important is that *letting* nature take its course is often advisable. Sometimes, and increasingly often, physicians initiate the discussion of letting nature take its course with patients and families; more often, families insist that all available measures be taken to sustain life, even against patients' wishes and physicians' advice. But it's also common for attending physicians to avoid mention of allowing a fatal condition to run its course,[8] and it must be explicitly requested by patients and/or their families.[9]

Society takes clinicians' mandate as one to preserve and enhance life when possible.[10] Now that it's become possible to technologically sustain life, that mandate has been automatically—we might say unthinkingly—extended to include the new ways of preserving life. Clinicians are given very limited discretion regarding *not* exercising their new capacity. Explicit notice is required, such as do-not-resuscitate orders.[11] But while the authority to decide against preserving life is acknowledged to rest with patients or, if they're incapacitated, with next of kin or surrogates, in practice, there is significant resistance on the part of many clinicians to withholding or withdrawing treatment[12] when doing so causes death.[13] The result is that the newly gained capacity for deciding death's timing poses an issue that is no longer only medical; it is now social and cultural, extending well beyond the boundaries of any single profession.

As soon as people dying at a particular time became more a matter of some*one's* decision rather than of some*thing's* consequences, the need arose for a communal coming to terms with the fact that we are increasingly faced with the need to make decisions about death's occurrence. The issue that needs communal resolution can be put quite simply: If we allow hospitalized, wholly dependent people to refuse treatment, and thus forfeit their lives to some underlying pathological condition or combination of conditions, shouldn't we allow and enable those same patients to decide whether death should be actively hastened?[14] One might ask why it's necessary to go this further step to assisted suicide,[15] why it isn't enough to refuse treatment.[16] This is a question that can be asked only by someone innocent of the nature of most terminal conditions, or by someone fully committed to an overriding moral or religious principle regarding suicide. The obvious answer is that dying "naturally" from terminal illness can be agonizing. When treatment is withheld or withdrawn, patients can linger for considerable periods. Even if their physical pain can be controlled, the process of dying can be utterly demeaning.

A major difficulty in resolving the question of whether assisted suicide is a natural and acceptable extension of refusal of treatment is that public debate of new challenges isn't usually as well directed as it might be. Public debate never seems to get things quite right. As the present debate over assisted suicide shows, while social response to medicine's new power has focused properly on the right to determine the timing of one's own death, the question has been framed and addressed too narrowly in terms of the common understanding of suicide. That is, the operant conception of suicide in the minds of the public is of willful relinquishment of life as a free choice. But suicide in the cases that concern us is a free choice only in the limited sense that it can be *autonomous*; it isn't a free choice in the ordinary sense because of a high degree of contextual coercion. To clarify, consider that individuals who kill themselves to avoid penury or criminal conviction[17] do so because they choose not to live as paupers or felons. Short of someone facing the death penalty, their suicides end viable lives. But those who choose to commit assisted suicide in the cases that concern us are people who are dying anyway. Their problem is that they are dying too slowly, and often too painfully. Their suicides only hasten deaths that are not only inevitable, in that we're all mortal, but also imminent and anticipated in all the detail that medical knowledge and experience can provide. This is a point that is too often glossed or ignored in debating assisted suicide in medical contexts.

The main reason for inadequately weighting the imminence of death in cases of assisted suicide is that given the value we place on life, we are strongly inclined to see willfully relinquishing artificially supported life just as we see willfully relinquishing viable life—i.e., as full-fledged suicide. We are concept-poor with regard to death in the new context defined by greater control over death's timing. The result is that we are making the concept of suicide do too much work to cover quite disparate sorts of cases.[18] We need finer-grained ways of describing what people do when they willingly succumb to delayed but inevitable death by requesting cessation of technological life support. We need better ways to describe what people do when they choose to relinquish lives that are in any case forfeit, in anticipation of hopeless suffering. These decisions and actions contrast with what people do when they choose to die for reasons having little or nothing to do with extreme deterioration of their bodies. We also need to differentiate between what people do when they help others curtail the prolongation of their dying, as opposed to what they do when they—usually wrongly—help others end their viable lives.[19]

Adding to the confusion is that some clinicians, vividly aware of their patients' conditions and of the consequences of withholding or withdrawing life support, see requesting cessation of treatment as suicide. As we noted in chapter 4,[20] many clinicians take the request for cessation of treatment as the suicidal act. This is a problematic point that generates two plausible but complex positions. One is that requested cessation of treatment is suicide on the patient's part and assisted suicide on the clinician's part. The other position is that requested cessation of treatment is voluntary euthanasia for both the patient and clinician involved.[21] The main arguments for the first position are that given patients' dependent situations, participating clinicians act as their agents. As we mentioned before, cessation of treatment then falls under Beauchamp's condition that "death is caused by conditions arranged by the person for the purpose of bringing about his or her own death."[22] Arguments for the second position, that cessation of treatment is voluntary euthanasia, turn on the fact that the patient does nothing other than making the actual request, that it is the involved clinician who takes the necessary steps, and that the real cause of death is the underlying condition and not the removal of the relevant life support.[23] Additionally, it's argued that it isn't always the case that cessation of life-support treatment results in death.[24]

A good deal turns on the question of whether cessation of treatment is more properly assisted suicide or voluntary euthanasia. There are tricky moral questions to be resolved. For example, if a patient's moral or religious beliefs prohibit suicide, and the patient requests cessation of treatment, is the patient deemed to be committing (assisted) suicide or only to be accepting (voluntary) euthanasia? Is the patient initiating a self-destructive sequence of events, or more innocently acquiescing to the hastening of the inevitable? Is the participating clinician merely implementing the patient's instructions, or performing a more direct act of taking life? And philosophical or moral considerations aside, the question of the degree of responsibility borne by a participating clinician could be crucial in a legal setting.

In general, individuals who are hospitalized with terminal conditions, or because of advanced age's debility, are people whose lives are being prolonged. Given modern medicine's capabilities, even fairly minimal hospital treatment of those individuals is life-prolonging. But in some cases, what is going on is that dying is being protracted. Moreover, without explicit contrary requests, the dying process most likely will continue to be protracted in many cases, despite increasing difficulty and recourse to more elaborate measures. Clinicians' professional responsibility and default practice are still to sustain life as long as is at least practically possible.[25] So far, patients' counterbalancing prerogatives have been largely limited to refusal of initiation of life-sustaining treatment or requested cessation of such treatment. But as current debate makes abundantly clear, attitudes toward the protraction of dying are changing. Many now think that once people are moribund, once they are dying of a pathological condition or because of their age, they ought to have the right not only to refuse treatment but also to more actively hasten their deaths. However, we're a long way from an obvious consensus on the question.

PRINCIPLES IN CONFLICT

Because clinicians acquired their new measure of control over death's occurrence gradually, through ongoing medical research and improved practice, it's assumed that the new capacity to keep patients alive longer is no different in principle from the capacity to treat their diseases or relieve their pain. This assumption leads naturally to another, which is that exercise of the new control is adequately governed by existing principles and professional ethics. The result is that many believe that regulation of aid in dying, whether assisted suicide, voluntary euthanasia, or simple cessation of treatment, is and should remain a medical matter.[26] What is likely to prevent aid in dying remaining a purely medical matter is that as clinical control over the timing of death increases, it becomes possible, and perhaps likely, for two of medicine's governing principles to conflict with a third principle. The principles of nonmaleficence and beneficence may clash with the principle of autonomy or respect for persons' free choices.

The conflict of principles can happen in at least two ways. Clinicians, now able to exercise greater control over patients' deaths, are inclined to understand nonmaleficence and beneficence as requiring that patients be kept alive as long as possible. "Doing no harm" is taken to mean "not letting die," and certainly "not killing." "Bringing about good" is taken to mean "keeping people alive." One sort of conflict, then, the more familiar one, is when clinicians interpret these principles as requiring them to prolong patients' lives despite some patients disagreeing that it's in their interests to be kept alive. The other, newer con flict is that a change in the interpretation of medicine's governing principles may prompt clinicians to take it on themselves to decide for their patients that it isn't in their interests to be kept alive, despite some patients being at least ambivalent about relinquishing life. Reinterpretation of the principles of beneficence and nonmaleficence as requiring that life not be unproductively sustained could contravene patients' autonomy as much as keeping them alive against their will. As we've said before, it isn't that clinicians are going to start killing their patients; it's that new perceptions may prompt them to discount patients' ambivalence or lack of readiness.

If all we needed to do was empower patients to receive requested assistance in suicide or voluntary euthanasia, the problem might be manageable. We already accept that patients may refuse treatment, so we would need only to work for the passage of appropriate legislation regarding assisted suicide and voluntary euthanasia. This is, in fact, how things look to many now. Admittedly, there's the additional need to train clinicians to appreciate that nonmaleficence and beneficence don't always require the preservation of life or the prolongation of dying, but that, too, might be manageable. However, empowering patients to choose assisted suicide or voluntary euthanasia means further empowering clinicians regarding the timing of death. This raises the possibilities we've considered, namely, of clinicians too readily acceding to requests for assistance in suicide or voluntary euthanasia, or paternalistically influencing patients to make such requests.

The practice of medicine has been conceived, at least since Hippocrates, as forbidding the doing of harm, interpreted as the causing of suffering and loss of life, and requiring the doing of good, interpreted as relieving or preventing suffering and preserving life. However, clinicians have always known that relieving or preventing greater suffering sometimes requires *not* preserving life, and some act accordingly. When they do, they do so believing that the principle of beneficence occasionally overrides the appearance of maleficence, as when aiding or causing death is the only way to relieve or prevent extreme suffering. Now, given the capacity to delay natural death significantly, we find ourselves needing to acknowledge and regularize clinicians' occasional and largely covert compassionate provision of aid in dying. The pressing question is what this will do to the practice of medicine. But as was noted earlier, the deeper issue is how we may be changing ourselves, especially those of us who become clinicians. We could be in the process of exalting "life that can be lived autonomously" and consequently "depreciating . . . life that is dependent."[27] We don't know how the practice of medicine will be affected if assisted suicide and voluntary euthanasia become conventionally available treatment options. In particular, we don't know if we can rely on those options being exercised only at the autonomous requests of patients. This concern has two aspects: first, the degree to which patients are capable of making autonomous decisions under the conditions in which suicide or euthanasia are appropriate, and second, the extent to which clinicians may unduly influence patients' decisions.[28]

We've already begun to change with respect to the maintenance of problematic life. At its simplest, the basic shift has been from the idea that "the more life the better" to a more complex recognition that life has a natural terminus and that delaying that terminus may be a profoundly unwise thing to do.[29] Experience with the ultimately pointless[30] technological maintenance of life has convinced many ethicists and clinicians that good medical practice doesn't always require such maintenance at great cost,[31] and that traditional medical practice too often prolongs life counterproductively. This change in view is perhaps most evident in what has been alluded to here and in previous chapters—namely, that ethicists and clinicians now think not in terms of unwarranted prolongation of *life* but in terms of unwarranted protraction of *dying*.[32] The traditional conception of caring for patients as people whose lives are threatened has changed to the conception of caring for some patients as people who have entered a final phase of life that may be wisely or unwisely prolonged. Putting this differently, a significant number of clinicians have gone from seeing death as always being a medical failure to seeing death as involving medical care only in the avoidance of unnecessary suffering.

This shift in perspective may be the maturing of professional attitudes that were unrealistically skewed when it became possible to clinically thwart death, if only for a time. But however salutary the shift, it could prompt practices at least as contrary to patient interests as the unwarranted prolongation of life. Just as protracting dying may be paternalistic contravention of patients' autonomy, too-ready accession to requests for assisted suicide or voluntary euthanasia and undue influencing of patients' suicidal or euthanasic decisions are also unacceptable paternalistic contraventions of autonomy. This is the threat prompting the slippery slope argument. It's perfectly possible that if assisted suicide is socially and professionally accepted, and possibly legalized, some clinicians will put budgetary considerations or institutional agendas above the interests of their patients. However, it's far more likely that the current conservative, life-sustaining paternalism that tends to predominate in medical practice may be replaced with a death-hastening paternalism.

The deepest part of the danger in clinicians adopting a death-hastening perspective on caring for terminal, very aged, and severely disabled patients is that patients will become complicitous in the possible contravention of their own interests. This may happen if our society as a whole adopts a different perspective on life. Our society may come to feel that "the older and disabled who are expensive should do *the responsible thing*."[33] From our present perspective, this possibility is deplorable, but a broad enough societal change of values could redefine what is right and wrong regarding those whose lives become problematic because of illness, age-related debility, or severe disability.[34] If that happens, the wholly dependent will enter hospitals and hospices with very different expectations; they'll be compliant to the undue influences and quick accession to requests for assisted suicide that we've discussed.[35]

Society has always asked a great deal from clinicians. The average person seems to think that anyone working in health care should show a devotion approaching selflessness. When one is grievously sick, there is little propensity to think of the welfare of others, and clinicians must bear the brunt of this forced self-absorption. Now we are asking clinicians to carry an even heavier burden. We are asking them to help us to relinquish our lives when those lives become unbearable. But we're also asking them to be judicious in acceding to our requests, knowing that we can't be altogether trusted to know what is best for us. And we're asking these things just when clinicians are being squeezed by economic pressures and by a substantial and escalating increase in the number of patients most likely to make these extra demands. To make things worse, we're asking these things when the profession is torn by ethically,[36] morally, and religiously driven disputes about the rightness of suicide and assisted suicide.

It's not surprising that clinicians are inclined to deal with these dismaying demands by resisting the complication of trying to meet them with more theory about how they should be met. But what is ultimately at risk, if theory and practice aren't reconciled regarding the provision of assisted suicide, aren't only unwarranted deaths and malpractice suits; what's at risk is our humanity. Those of us who care for the dying must learn to appreciate the force and necessity of universal principles as much as we are moved by the particular and contextual. Decisions about particular cases must be informed by general requirements. Though blindness to clinical particulars renders ethical theory irrelevant to what it should govern, impatience with preconditional abstractions indentures clinical practice to the emotional and the political. We face a tremendously difficult challenge posed by our new ability to delay our deaths, and it's in the form of recurring dilemmas calling for balanced assessments and responses. In choosing to practice rational assisted suicide and voluntary euthanasia, we seek to avoid two extremes. One is dehumanizing ourselves by using technology to turn people into bodies living well after everything that makes them persons has disappeared. The other is dehumanizing ourselves by depreciating "the life that is dependent"[37] and letting compassionate aid in dying degenerate into "the attractive solution of first resort."[38] There aren't any set answers to the question of when it's best to let life go; we have to repeatedly achieve a difficult equilibrium between reason's requirements and compassion's demands. Regrettably, the burden of achieving this equilibrium falls mainly on clinicians, because it is they who deal with those who might best let their lives go. Ethical theorists can help by learning to be more sensitive to the realities of what they theorize about, but clinicians need to learn that technology has forever changed the practice of medicine by making ethical theory as intrinsic to it as knowledge of anatomy. The prospects of adding difficult work in ethical theory to the already overwhelming medical curriculum are daunting, but we face a tremendous challenge. As Sandel puts it,

> [e]ven those who regard life as a sacred trust can admit that the claims of compassion may sometimes override the duty to preserve life. The challenge is to find a way to honor these claims that preserves the moral burden of hastening death, and that retains the reverence for life as something we cherish, not something we choose.[39]

It's not surprising that clinicians are inclined to resist theoretical complication of this challenge, or that theoreticians are inclined to think that formulation of clear principles should suffice to meet it. But each group needs to meet the other halfway. What is ultimately at risk, if theory and practice can't be better reconciled on assisted suicide, aren't just unwarranted deaths and malpractice suits—it's our humanity. Assisted suicide is done now and will likely be done considerably more in the future. We can't afford to let it degenerate into "the attractive solution of first resort."[40]

NOTES

1. Mydans 1997; emphasis added.

2. Mydans 1997.

3. In fact, there's a sense in which the meaning or force of *natural* is now simply *untreated*.

4. Kübler-Ross 1969; see chapter 2.

5. By this we mean the fives of those who have terminal illnesses, those who are so severely disabled that they can't survive without fairly intensive and continuous care, and those whose advanced age has made them wholly dependent on others.

6. We have to remember that for the great bulk of human history, it fell on families—usually the women—to look after the dying. But now, most people of advanced age, with great debility, or with terminal conditions die in hospitals, nursing homes, or hospices. In short, the cost of their care falls largely on society.

7. Antibiotics wouldn't only be *decreased*, since that could simply add to patients' discomfort and still retard the underlying disease. Also, some uses of antibiotics in terminal cases only ease pain or discomfort without affecting the underlying disease. In some cases, keeping someone alive doesn't involve antibiotics or complex equipment at all. As simple a routine as periodically turning an immobile patient in bed prevents contraction of possibly fatal pneumonia by not allowing liquid to pool in the lungs and inviting infection.

8. Fein 1997a.

9. It may appear that since the Quinlan case in the United States and the Nancy B. case in Canada, such requests usually involve the courts. This is decidedly not the case. The great majority of decisions to withhold or cease treatment are made by attending physicians in concert with the patient and family. Those decisions usually don't even involve hospital administrators. It's only if there are special circumstances or the case is problematic that institutional or legal authorities become involved. The Quinlan and Nancy B. cases certainly set precedents for most clinicians, but they didn't establish legal procedures that have been routinely followed since then.

10. See, e.g., Pellegrino 1992.

11. Moreover, instructions such as do-not-resuscitate orders must be carefully followed. An order not to resuscitate a patient means just that; it doesn't admit of looser interpretation.

12. See Fein 1997a.

13. Some physicians, while acknowledging that it's the patient's prerogative to have treatment stopped, refuse to do so themselves, sometimes withdrawing from cases in which the request is made.

14. We don't say "and families or surrogates" here, because if patients are,

for whatever reasons, incapable of choosing to commit assisted suicide, it isn't enough to have attending clinicians and family make the decision. It may not be necessary to involve the courts, but minimally, some sort of independent or "arm's-length" board should assess the matter.

15. The question of voluntary euthanasia also arises, of course, but that is not our primary concern here.

16. See Callahan 1993, 1995.

17. Note that we aren't considering suicide done for irrational reasons, such as clinical depression or to be transported to an alien heaven.

18. It's simplistic to see requesting cessation of treatment as committing suicide simply because the anticipated consequence is death. There is an important conceptual difference between allowing someone to die, even if it is oneself, and killing someone, including oneself. The absence of practical difference makes many clinicians impatient with this—and other—distinctions, but overlooking the conceptual differences leads to overlooking attendant moral differences.

19. Just as clinical ethicists and clinicians have distinguished between prolonging life and prolonging the process of dying (Whytehead and Chidwick 1980:29), we need to distinguish between *taking* one's own life and *forfeiting* one's life to an underlying pathological condition or advanced age. Choosing to forfeit life is not quite self-destruction as suicide has been traditionally conceived. People in good health who shoot themselves certainly commit suicide, but while terminally ill people who ask to have life support stopped may be *choosing* to die, they commit suicide in a sense that needs qualification, if only to clarify the question of the responsibility borne by those who assist their suicides. The most obvious qualification has to do with the directness of the cause of death. Regardless of how sure patients and clinicians are that cessation of life support will prove fatal, it is still an assumption, albeit a strong one, that those whose treatment is stopped will die without the relevant drugs or apparatus. They may confound expectations and in fact live for a considerable period after cessation of treatment. This point was crucial in the fairly easy way that cessation of treatment was socially and legally accepted. But the qualification has little to do with chances of survival; it is, after all, possible that one might shoot oneself in the head and survive. The qualification has to do with straightforward causality.

20. See the section "A Question of Categorization."

21. We owe much of the point being made here to Russell R. Savage, an Alberta Crown prosecutor who took the time to clearly outline for us the opposed positions.

22. Beauchamp 1980:77, quoted in Rachels 1986:81.

23. CGP agrees strongly with this position, holding that cessation of treatment is the *removal* of a causal factor; to cease treating is to stop intervening in pathological and physiological chains of events. It's to allow a causal process that has been interrupted or retarded to continue. In contrast, shooting oneself or ingesting poison is *introduction* of a lethal causal factor. It is a matter of ini-

tiating a causal process. In the former case, life is forfeited to a pathological causal process by removing another causal process that counters the effects of the first; in the latter case, a causal process is begun to terminate life. Suicide, in the full sense, requires an agent-initiated direct cause of death. Neither a pathological condition nor advanced age is that sort of cause. If a person is dying because of a pathological condition or age and some sort of death-delaying treatment is being exercised, stopping that treatment is suicide only in the sense that life is forfeited to the underlying process. Life isn't *taken* by stopping treatment; life is taken by what the treatment inhibits or suspends. Moral and legal questions may turn on the difference, and we can't allow the fact that death is virtually certain upon the cessation of treatment to obscure the fact that suicide is *self-killing*.

24. For example, Karen Ann Quinlan survived in a vegetative state for nine years after being removed from a ventilator and body-temperature-controlling apparatus (see Stevens 1997).

25. Again, see Fein 1997a.

26. However, the matter of cessation of treatment effectively stopped being a purely medical issue with the 1976 Karen Ann Quinlan case. Previously, getting clinicians not to prolong life, against the interests and wishes of patients and families, was a matter of discussion among patients, family members, and attending clinicians, but the Quinlan case took the question of cessation of treatment to the courts. Once it became possible to sustain the life of even patients in vegetative states for long periods of time, stronger measures were required to counter the working medical assumption that life should be preserved as long as possible (see Stevens 1997).

27. Steinfels 1997a:12.

28. See Checkland and Silberfeld 1993, 1995, 1996; also Diegner and Sloan 1992.

29. SJT dealt with a patient who was quadriplegic, had had a tracheostomy, and subsequently had to be resuscitated three times, each time spending over a week in intensive care. The patient's suffering was controlled with difficulty, and there was also difficulty with communication. It was, in fact, unclear whether the patient was still competent. There was no question whatever of significant improvement. The strong likelihood was that several more resuscitations would follow and with greater frequency. In such cases, it seems the only thing that the use of technology to maintain life succeeds in doing is ensuring the need for *further* application of the same or even more elaborate technology. Unfortunately, "the public and legislative debates about dying with dignity and the rights of the terminally ill to hasten their own deaths have not caused meaningful discussions among doctors and patients, and patients and their loved ones, regarding treatment as death nears" (Fein 1997a).

30. Many who consider life an unrenounceable gift will reject this use of "pointless," because they believe that every moment of continued awareness is valuable in itself.

31. "Cost" here doesn't mean only the use of scarce resources and actual expense. It includes what patients whose lives are maintained must bear and what their families and friends must bear.

32. Whytehead and Chidwick 1980:29.

33. Interview with Arthur Caplan, "The Kevorkian Verdict," *Frontline*, broadcast May 14, 1996; our emphasis. As Battin has observed, "*suicide is cheap*" (Battin 1987:169; emphasis in original). The cost of caring for, or simply maintaining, elderly or severely disabled patients is alarming. If even 10 percent of those patients could be made to commit suicide in order to stop draining scarce medical resources, and thus denying those resources to more viable patients, the health-care system would realize substantial savings.

34. Our present worldview is largely—though often inconsistently—relativistic. As we've maintained ourselves, *rational* is not defined by a transcendental absolute but by communal consensus. In the same way, what now looks to be contravention of patient interests may become the established way of dealing with those interests. Relativism is essentially the view that "cognitive, moral, or aesthetic claims involving . . . truth, meaningfulness, rightness [and] reasonableness . . . are relative to the contexts in which they appear" (Krausz 1989:1). These contexts may be understood as social, cultural, professional, or even individual, but they are taken as what determines what is right and what is wrong. Still, at the same time, we experience communal outrage and are quick to invoke principle when our interests are directly affected. But what matters here is that in arguing against a perspective change regarding life maintenance, recourse to claimed objective and universal principles is no longer decisive. If anything, it's seen as privileging personal values.

In trying to understand how we took this Nietzschean turn, Rorty observes that the root of the change was something "glimpsed at the end of the eighteenth century," which was the momentous idea "that anything [can] . . . be made to look good or bad . . . by being redescribed" (Rorty 1989:7). This idea made it "possible, toward the end of the nineteenth century, to . . . juggle several descriptions . . . without asking which one was right" (Rorty 1989:39). The "juggling" of descriptions meant that rival redescriptions of something, as competing interpretations of principles, came to be considered not mutually exclusive competitors for unique correctness, but alternative accounts to be assessed relative to particular purposes and perspectives.

35. As CGP discusses elsewhere, patient compliance to undue influence and too-ready accession to assisted suicide won't be contravention of patients' autonomy, because the very concept of autonomy will have changed (*The Reduction of Dependent Life*, forthcoming).

36. Recall that we're using *ethical* to refer to professional codes of conduct.

37. Steinfels 1997a:12.

38. Caplan interview.

39. Sandel 1997:27.

40. Caplan interview.

BIBLIOGRAPHY

We've departed from scholarly tradition by including a significant number of references to media items, including newspaper articles and televised reports and interviews. Our aim is threefold: to avail ourselves of succinct, accessible commentaries on the issue; to reflect the considerable media attention being given the issue of assisted suicide; and to provide the most recent survey figures available. Media articles bearing their authors' names are listed in the "Books and Articles" section; anonymous media items are listed in the "Media" section.

BOOKS AND ARTICLES

Agee, James. 1985. *A Death in the Family*. New York: Bantam.

Alemayehu, E., D. Mooloy, G. Guyatt, J. Singer, et al. 1991. "Variability in Physicians' Decisions on Caring for Chronically Ill Elderly Patients: An International Study." *Canadian Medical Association Journal* 144(9): 1133–38.

Alther, Lisa. 1976. *Kinflicks*. London: Penguin.

Alvarez, Al. 1971. *The Savage God: A Study of Suicide*. New York: Penguin.

Anders, George. 1997. *Health Against Wealth: HMOs and the Breakdown of Medical Trust*. New York: Houghton Mifflin.

Angell, Marcia. 1997a. "Anguished Debate: Should Doctors Help Their Patients Die?" *New York Times*, June 24, 1997. (Excerpted from Angell 1997b.)

———. 1997b. "Editorials: The Supreme Court and Physician-assisted Suicide—the Ultimate Right." *New England Journal of Medicine* 336(1): 50–53.

———. 1990. "The Right to Die in Dignity." *Newsweek* 116 (July 23): 9.

Angier, Natalie. 1995. "Scientists Mull Role of Empathy in Man and Beast." *New York Times*, May 9.

Annas, G. J. 1991. "The Health Care Proxy and the Living Will." *New England Journal of Medicine* 324(17): 1210–13.

Appleby, Timothy. 1996. "Doctor Death Ignores Legalities in Mission of Mercy." *Globe and Mail*, May 9.

Appleby, Timothy, and Jill Mahoney. 1997. "MDs' Death Role: Murder or Mercy?" *Globe and Mail*, May 9.

Aries, Phillipe. 1982. *The Hour of Our Death*. Trans. Helen Weaver. New York: Vintage Books.

Artaud, Antonin. 1995. "On Suicide," in *Le Disque Vert* 1 (1925), quoted in *The Columbia Dictionary of Quotations*. 1995. New York: Columbia University Press, Microsoft *Bookshelf*, 1996–97 CD-ROM edition.

Ashby, M. 1994. "A Proposed Advance Directive Format for South Australia." *Australian Health Law Bulletin* 2(7): 89–92.

Ashton, G. 1994. *The Elderly Client Handbook—The Law Society's Guide to Acting for Older People*. London: Law Society.

Auclair, François, Jean Leroux, Anthony Weinberg, and Jeffrey Turnbull. 1996. "Logic in Medicine: A Need to Teach Avoidance of Fallacies." *Annals of the Royal College of Physicians and Surgeons of Canada* 30(2): 101–102.

Audi, Robert, ed. 1995. *The Cambridge Dictionary of Philosophy*. Cambridge: Cambridge University Press.

Ayer, Alfred J., and Jane O'Grady, eds. 1992. *A Dictionary of Philosophical Quotations*. Oxford: Blackwell.

Baechler, Jean. 1975. *Suicides*. Trans. Barry Cooper. New York: Basic Books.

Baird, Robert M., and Stuart E. Rosenbaum, eds. 1997. *Euthanasia: The Moral Issues*. Amherst, N.Y.: Prometheus Books.

Barry, Dan. 1997. "New York's Chief Lawyer Argues Suicide Case." *New York Times*, January 9.

Battin, Margaret Pabst. 1982. *Ethical Issues in Suicide*. Englewood Cliffs, N.J.: Prentice-Hall.

———. 1984. "The Concept of Rational Suicide." In *Death: Current Perspectives*. 3d ed. Ed. Edwin Shneidman. Mountain View, Calif.: Mayfield.

———. 1987. "Choosing the Time to Die: The Ethics and Economics of Suicide in Old Age," in *Ethical Dimensions of Geriatric Care*. Ed. Stuart Spicker, Stanley Ingman, and Ian Lawson. Dordrecht: Reidel.

———. 1990. *Ethics in the Sanctuary: Examining the Practices of Organized Religion*. New Haven, Conn.: Yale University Press.

————. 1991. "Euthanasia: The Way We Do It, the Way They Do It." *Journal of Pain and Symptom Management* 6(5): 298–305.

————. 1992a. "Assisted Suicide: Can We Learn Anything from Germany?" *Hastings Center Report* (March–April): 44–51.

————. 1992b. "Voluntary Euthanasia and the Risks of Abuse: Can We Learn Anything from the Netherlands?" *Law Medicine and Health Care* 20(1–2): 133–43.

————. 1994. *The Least Worst Death.* New York and Oxford: Oxford University Press.

————. 1995. *Ethical Issues in Suicide.* Englewood Cliffs, N.J.: Prentice-Hall. (Revised version of Battin 1982b.)

————. 1996. *The Death Debate: Ethical Issues in Suicide.* Englewood Cliffs, N.J.: Prentice-Hall. (This is the same work as Battin 1995, with a foreword by Dr. Timothy Quill and repaginated.)

Battin, Margaret Pabst, and Arthur G. Lipman. 1996. *Drug Use in Assisted Suicide and Euthanasia.* New York: Pharmaceutical Products Press.

Battin, Margaret Pabst, and D. J. Mayo, eds. 1980. *Suicide: The Philosophical Issues.* New York: St. Martin's Press.

Bayda, Edward. 1995. "Is Robert Latimer's Life Sentence 'Cruel and Unusual Punishment'? The Sentence Is 'Grossly Disproportionate.'" *Globe and Mail,* July 20.

Bayer, Ronald, Daniel Callahan, John Fletcher, et al. 1983. "The Care of the Terminally Ill: Morality and Economics." *New England Journal of Medicine* 309: 1490–94.

Baylis, Françoise, Jocelyn Downie, Benjamin Freedman, Barry Hoffmaster, and Susan Sherwin, eds. 1995. *Health Care Ethics in Canada.* Toronto: Harcourt Brace.

Beauchamp, Tom L. 1980. "Suicide." In *Matters of Life and Death.* Ed. Tom Regan. Philadelphia: Temple University Press.

————. 1996. *Intending Death: The Ethics of Assisted Suicide and Euthanasia.* Upper Saddle River, N.J.: Prentice-Hall.

Beauchamp, Tom L., ed. 1975. *Ethics and Public Policy.* Englewood Cliffs, N.J.: Prentice-Hall.

Beauchamp, Tom L., and James Childress. 1994. *Principles of Biomedical Ethics,* 4th ed. Oxford: Oxford University Press.

Beauchamp, Tom L., and Seymour Perlin, eds. 1978. *Ethical Issues In Death and Dying.* Englewood Cliffs, N.J.: Prentice-Hall.

Beauchamp, Tom L., and LeRoy Walters. 1989. *Contemporary Issues in Bioethics,* 3rd ed. Belmont, Calif.: Wadsworth Publishing Company.

Benjamin, Martin, and Joy Curtis. 1986. *Ethics in Nursing.* Oxford: Oxford University Press.

Bennahum, D., G. Kimsma, C. Spreeuwenberg, et al. 1993. "Been There: Physicians Speak for Themselves." *Cambridge Quarterly of Healthcare Ethics* 2: 9–17.

Benrubi, Guy. 1992. "Euthanasia—The Need for Procedural Safeguards." *New England Journal of Medicine* 326(3): 197–99.

Berger, David M. 1987. *Clinical Empathy*. Northvale, N.J.: Aronson.

Berke, Richard L. 1997. "The Nation: Suddenly, the New Politics of Morality." *New York Times*, June 15.

Betzold, Michael. 1993. *Appointment with Dr. Death*. Troy, Mich.: Momentum Books.

Biggs, H., and K. Diesfeld. 1995. "Assisted Suicide for People with Depression: An Advocate's Perspective." *Medical Law International* 2: 23–37.

Birren, James E. 1968. "Psychological Aspects of Aging: Intellectual Functioning." *Gerontologist* 8:16–19.

Birren, James E., and K. Warner Schaie, eds. 1977. *Handbook of the Psychology of Aging*. New York: Van Nostrand.

Bix, B. 1995. "Physician Assisted Suicide and the United States Constitution." *Modern Law Review* 58(3): 404–11.

Bliss, Michael. 1990. "What Price Immortality?" *Report on Business Magazine*, *Globe and Mail*, August.

Blustein, Jeffrey. 1993. "The Family in Medical Decisionmaking." *Hastings Center Report* 23(3): 6–14.

Blythe, Ronald. 1979. *The View in Winter*. New York: Harcourt Brace Jovanovich.

Bond, E. J. 1988. " 'Good' and 'Good for': A Reply to Hurka." *Mind* 97: 279–80.

———. 1996. *Ethics and Human Well-Being*. Oxford: Blackwell.

Bonsteel, Alan. 1997. "Behind the White Coat." *Humanist* 57(2): 15–18.

Boswell, James. 1947. "An Account of My Last Interview with David Hume, Esq." Appendix A to *Hume's Dialogues Concerning Natural Religion*, by Norman Kemp Smith. 2d ed. London: Thomas Nelson and Sons.

Botwinick, Jack. 1967. *Cognitive Processes in Maturity and Old Age*. New York: Springer.

Bradsher, Keith. 1997. "Kevorkian Is Also Painter. His Main Theme Is Death." *New York Times*, March 17.

Brandt, R. B. 1975. "The Morality and Rationality of Suicide." In *A Handbook for the Study of Suicide*. Ed. Seymour Perlin. Oxford: Oxford University Press.

Bresnahan James F. 1993. "Medical Futility or the Denial of Death?" *Cambridge Quarterly of Healthcare Ethics* 2(2): 213–17.

Brewster, Murray. 1998. "Doctor Could Face Manslaughter Charge: Nova Scotia Attorney General Wants Clearer Guidelines on When Patients' Lives Can Be Terminated." *Globe and Mail*, July 3.

Brickman, Harriet. 1995. "Live and Let Die: A Doctor's Best Hopes Can Be a Patient's Worst Nightmare." *New York Times Magazine*, July 2.

British Medical Association. 1988. *Euthanasia*. London: BMA.

———. 1993. *Medical Ethics Today*. London: BMA.

Brock, Dan. 1986. "Forgoing Life-Sustaining Food and Water: Is It Killing?" In

By No Extraordinary Means. Ed. Joanne Lynn. Bloomington and Indianapolis: Indiana University Press.

———. 1989. "Death and Dying." In *Medical Ethics.* Ed. Robert M. Veatch. Boston: Jones and Bartlett.

———. 1995. "Voluntary Active Euthanasia." In *Health Care Ethics in Canada.* Ed. Françoise Baylis et al. Toronto: Harcourt Brace.

Brodie, Howard. 1976. *Ethical Decisions in Medicine.* Boston: Little, Brown.

Brody, Jane E. 1997. "Personal Health: When a Dying Patient Seeks Suicide Aid, It May Be a Signal to Fight Depression." *New York Times,* June 18.

Brody, H. 1992. "Assisted Death—A Compassionate Response to a Medical Failure." *New England Journal of Medicine* 327(19): 1384–88.

Bromley, D. B. 1974. *The Psychology of Human Aging.* London: Penguin.

Brooks, Simon A. 1984. "Dignity and Cost-Effectiveness: A Rejection of the Utilitarian Approach to Death." *Journal of Medical Ethics* 10:148–51.

Brown, Newell. 1986. *How Not to Overstay One's Life: To Call It a Day—In Good Season.* Nederland, Colo.: Privately published. (Available from Newell Brown, Twin Sisters Road, Magnolia Star Route, Nederland, CO 80466.)

Bruni, Frank. 1996. "Court Overturns Ban in New York on Aided Suicides: A Historic Shift, Federal Ruling Allows Doctors to Prescribe Drugs to End Life." *New York Times,* April 3.

———. 1997. "Leader Believed in Space Aliens and Apocalypse." *New York Times,* March 28.

Bullock, A., O. Stallybrass, and S. Trombley, eds. 1988. *The Fontana Dictionary of Modern Thought.* London: Fontana.

Burgess, J. A. 1993. "The Great Slippery-Slope Argument." *Journal of Medical Ethics* 19: 169–74.

Caine, Eric. 1993. "Self-Determined Death, the Physician, and Medical Priorities: Is There Time To Talk?" *Journal of the American Medical Association* 270(7): 875–76.

Callahan, Daniel. 1993. "Pursuing a Peaceful Death." *Hastings Center Report* 23(4): 33–38.

———. 1995. "When Self-Determination Runs Amok." In *Health Care Ethics in Canada.* Ed. Françoise Baylis et al. Toronto: Harcourt Brace.

Campbell, Murray. 1991. "Voters Get Say on Right to Die." *Globe and Mail,* October 21.

Campbell, Robert, and Diane Collinson. 1988. *Ending Lives.* Oxford: Basil Blackwell.

Campi, Christina Walker. 1998. "When Dying Is as Hard as Birth." *New York Times,* January 5.

Camus, Albert. 1955. *The Myth of Sisyphus and Other Essays.* Trans. J. O'Brien. New York: Knopf.

Caplan, Arthur. 1981. "The 'Unnaturalness' of Aging—A Sickness Unto Death?" In *Concepts of Health and Disease.* Ed. Arthur Caplan, H. Tristram Engelhardt Jr., and James J. McCartney. Reading, Mass.: Addison-Wesley.

Caplan, Arthur, H. Tristram Engelhardt Jr., and James J. McCartney, eds. 1981. *Concepts of Health and Disease*. Reasing, Mass.: Addison-Wesley.

Capron, Alexander Morgan. 1986. "Legal and Ethical Problems in Decisions for Death." *Law, Medicine and Health Care* 14(3–4): 141–44, 157.

———. 1992. "The Patient Self-Determination Act: A Cooperative Model for Implementation." *Cambridge Quarterly of Healthcare Ethics* 1(2): 97–106.

Caralis, P. V. 1993. "The Influence of Ethnicity and Race on Attitudes Toward Advance Directives, Life-Prolonging Treatments, and Euthanasia." *Journal of Clinical Ethics* 4(2): 155–65.

Carpenter, B. 1993. "A Review and New Look at Ethical Suicide in Advanced Age." *Gerontologist* 33(3): 359–65.

Carter, Stephen L. 1996. "Rush to Lethal Judgment." *New York Times Magazine* (July 21): 28–29.

Cassell, Eric J. 1980. *The Healer's Art*. New York: Penguin Books.

———. 1991. *The Nature of Suffering and the Goals of Medicine*. New York: Oxford University Press.

Chappell P., and R. King. 1992. "Final Exit and the Risk of Suicide." *Journal of the American Medical Association* 267(22): 3027.

Checkland, David, and Michel Silberfeld. 1993. "Competence and the Three A's: Autonomy, Authenticity, and Aging." *Canadian Journal on Aging* 12(4): 453–68.

———. 1995. "Reflections on Segregating and Assessing Areas of Competence." *Theoretical Medicine* 16: 375–88.

———. 1996. "Mental Competence and the Question of Beneficent Intervention." *Theoretical Medicine* 17:121–34.

Childress, James F. 1979. "Paternalism and Health Care." In *Medical Responsibility*. Eds. Wade L. Robinson and Michael S. Pritchard. Clifton, N.J.: Humana Press.

Choice in Dying, Inc. 1991. *Refusal of Treatment Legislation—A State by State Compilation of Enacted and Model Statutes*. New York: Choice in Dying.

Choron, Jacques. 1963. *Death and Western Thought*. London: Collier-Macmillan.

———. 1972. *Suicide*. New York: Scribners.

Christakis, N., and D. Asch. 1993. "Biases in How Physicians Choose to Withdraw Life Support." *Lancet* 342:642–46.

Ciesielski-Carlucci, C. 1993. "Physician Attitudes and Experiences with Assisted Suicide: Results of a Small Opinion Survey." *Cambridge Quarterly of Healthcare Ethics* 2:39–44.

Ciesielski-Carlucci, C., and G. Kimsma. 1994. "The Impact of Reporting Cases of Euthanasia in Holland: A Patient and Family Perspective." *Bioethics* 8(2): 151–58.

Clark, Nina. 1997. *The Politics of Physician Assisted Suicide*. New York: Garland.

Code, Lorraine. 1991. *What Can She Know?: Feminist Theory and the Construction of Knowledge*. Ithaca, N.Y.: Cornell University Press.

———. 1994. "I Know Just How You Feel." In *The Empathic Practitioner*. Eds. Ellen Singer More and Maureen A. Milligan. New Brunswick, N.J.: Rutgers University.

Cohen, Roger. 1997. "2 'Perfect Little Girls' Stun France in Suicide." *New York Times*, May 30.

Colt, George Howe. 1991. *The Enigma of Suicide*. New York: Summit Books.

Conwell, Yeates, and Eric Caine. 1991. "Rational Suicide and the Right to Die—Reality and Myth." *New England Journal of Medicine* 325(15): 1100–1103.

Coutts, Jane. 1997. "HMOs: Health Service or Horror Show?" *Globe and Mail*, April 19.

Coutts, Jane, and Henry Hess. 1996. "Doctor Charged in Man's Suicide," *Globe and Mail*, June 21.

Cowley, Malcolm. 1982. *The View from Eighty*. London: Penguin.

Cox, Donald. 1993. *Hemlock's Cup: The Struggle for Death With Dignity*. Amherst, N.Y.: Prometheus Books.

Cox, Kevin. 1997a. "Doctor Charged with Murder." *Globe and Mail*, May 8.

———. 1997b. "Families Wondering If Relatives Killed." *Globe and Mail*, May 9.

———. 1998a. "Crown Wants Morrison Case to Proceed: Ruling in Patient's Death 'Bad in Law.'" *Globe and Mail*, June 6.

———. 1998b. "Murder Charge Against Halifax Doctor Dismissed: Discharge Reopens Issue of Treating Dying Patients." *Globe and Mail*, February 28.

Crisp, R. 1987. "A Good Death: Who Best to Bring It?" *Bioethics* 1(1): 74–79.

———. 1994. "Reasonable Care? Some Comments on Gillett's Reasonable Care." *Bioethics* 8(2): 159–67.

Crowley, J. 1992. "To Be or Not to Be: Examining the Right to Die." *Journal of Legislation of Notre Dame Law School* 18(2): 347–55.

Dao, James. 1996. "Suicide Ruling Raises Concern: Who Decides?" *New York Times*, April 4.

Daube, David. 1972. "The Linguistics of Suicide." *Philosophy and Public Affairs* 1: 387–437.

Davis, A., L. Phillips, T. Drought, et al. 1995. "Nurses' Attitudes Towards Active Euthanasia." *Nursing Outlook* 43(4): 174–79.

Day, M. 1994. "An Act of Will." *Nursing Times* 90(10): 14.

de Beauvoir, Simone. 1969. *A Very Easy Death*. Harmondsworth: Penguin Books.

De Spelder, Lynne Ann, and Albert Lee Strickland. 1992. *The Last Dance: Encountering Death and Dying*, 3d ed. Mountain View, Calif.: Mayfield.

Degrazia, David. 1995. "Value Theory and the Best Interests Standard." *Bioethics* 9(1): 50–61.

Delden J, P. Maas, L. Pijnenborg, and C. Looman. 1993. "Deciding Not to Resuscitate in Dutch Hospitals." *Journal of Medical Ethics* 19: 200–205.

Delden J., L. Pijnenborg, and P. Maas. 1993a. "Dances With Data." *Bioethics* 7: 323–29.

———. 1993b. "The Remmelink Study: Two Years Later." *Hastings Center Report* 23(6): 24–27.

DeSimone, Cathleen. 1996. *Death on Demand: Physician-assisted Suicide in the United States*. Buffalo, N.Y.: W. S. Hein.

Devettere, Raymond J. 1992. "Slippery Slopes and Moral Reasoning." *Journal of Clinical Ethics* 3(4): 297–301.

Dickens, Bernard. 1993. "A Response to the Papers of Molloy and Colleagues (Canada) and Cranford (United States) on Advance Directives." *Humane Medicine* 9(1):78–84.

Diegner, Leslie F., and Jeffrey Sloan. 1992. "Decision-Making During Serious Illness: What Role Do Patients Really Want To Play?" *Clinical Epidemiology* 45(9): 941–50.

Doerr, Edd. 1997. "Liberty and Death." *Humanist* 57(2): 12–13.

Donnelly, John, ed. 1978. *Language, Metaphysics, and Death*. New York: Fordham University Press.

———. 1997. *Suicide: Right or Wrong?* Amherst, N.Y.: Prometheus Books.

Donnie, J., G. Gopalakrishnan, et al. 1995. "The Relationship of Empathy to Moral Reasoning in First Year Medical Students." *Cambridge Quarterly of Healthcare Ethics* 4: 448–53.

Downey, Donn. 1992. "Waiting for That Final Visitor." *Globe and Mail*, April 8.

Downie, R. S. 1994. "Limiting Treatment at the End of Life." *VESS Newsletter* (January): 1–3.

Downie, R. S., and K. Calman. 1994. *Healthy Respect: Ethics in Health Care*. Oxford: Oxford University Press.

Downing, A. B., ed. 1969. *Euthanasia and the Right to Death: The Case for Voluntary Euthanasia*. Atlantic Highlands, N.J.: Humanities Press.

Doyal, Len, and Daniel Wilsher. 1993. "Withholding Cardiopulmonary Resuscitation: Proposals for Formal Guidelines." *British Medical Journal* 306: 1593–96.

Dresser, R., and P. Whitehouse. 1994. "The Incompetent Patient on the Slippery Slope." *Hastings Center Report* 24(4): 6–12.

Drey, P., and J. Giszczak. 1992. "May I Author My Final Chapter? Assisted Suicide and Guidelines to Prevent Abuse." *Journal of Legislation of the Notre Dame Law School* 18(2): 331–45.

Dreyfus, Hubert, and Paul Rabinow. 1983. *Michel Foucault: Beyond Structuralism and Hermeneutics*. With an Afterword by Michel Foucault. Brighton, England: Harvester Press.

Durkheim, Emile. [1897] 1951. *Suicide: A Study in Sociology*. Trans. J. A. Spaulding and G. Simpson. New York: Free Press.

Dworkin, Gerald. 1972. "Paternalism." *Monist* 56 (January): 76f.

Dworkin, Ronald. 1993. *Life's Dominion—An Argument About Abortion and Euthanasia*. London: HarperCollins.

———. 1994. "When Is It Right to Die?" *New York Times*, May, 17.

———. 1996. "Sex, Death, and the Courts." *New York Review of Books* 43(13): 44–50.

Dworkin, Ronald, et al. 1997. "Assisted Suicide: The Philosophers' Brief." *New York Review of Books* 44(5): 41–47.

Edwards, Paul, ed. 1967. *The Encyclopedia of Philosophy*, Vol. 4. New York: Macmillan and Free Press.

Egan, Timothy. 1998. "First Death Under Assisted-Suicide Law: Moving a Debate from the Abstract to the Actual." *New York Times*, March 26.

———. 1997. "Assisted Suicide Comes Full Circle, to Oregon." *New York Times*, October 26.

Emanuel Ezekiel, and Linda Emanuel. 1992. "Proxy Decision Making for Incompetent Patients: An Ethical and Empirical Analysis." *Journal of the American Medical Association* 267(15): 2067–71.

———. 1993. "Decisions at the End of Life Guided by Communities of Patients." *Hastings Center Report* (September–October) 6–14.

———. 1997. "Assisted Suicide? Not in My State," *New York Times*, July 24.

Emanuel, Linda, M. Barry, J. Stoeckle, et al. 1991. "Advance Directives for Medical Care—A Case for Greater Use." *New England Journal of Medicine* 324(13): 889–95.

Emanuel, Ezekiel, Linda Emanuel, J. Stoeckle, L. Hummel, and M. Barry. 1994. "Advance Directives: Stability of Patients' Treatment Choices." *Archives of Internal Medicine* 154: 209–17.

Evans, D., H. Funkenstein, M. Albert, P. Scherr, et al. 1989. "Prevalence of Alzheimer's Disease in a Community Population of Older Persons: Higher than Previously Reported." *Journal of the American Medical Association* 262(18): 2551–56.

Farbar, Jennifer. 1995. "Hush of Suicide," *New York Times Magazine*, March 5.

Farber, Leslie H. 1969. "The Phenomenology of Suicide." In *On the Nature of Suicide*. Ed. Edwin Shneidman. San Francisco: Jossey-Bass.

Farr, Moira. 1997. "When Mr. D Calls, Get Ready to Dance." *Globe and Mail*, April 19.

Feifel, Herman, ed. 1977. *New Meanings of Death*. New York: McGraw-Hill.

Fein, Esther B. 1996. "Court Overturns Ban in New York on Aided Suicides: The Decision Offers Relief to Plaintiffs," *New York Times*, April 3.

———. 1997a. "A Better Quality of Life, in the Days Before Death." *New York Times*, May 4.

———. 1997b. "Handling of Assisted-Suicide Cases Unlikely to Shift, Officials Say." *New York Times*, June 27.

———. 1997c. "Not Dead Enough to Die: Laws Force Life Support on a Man Who Never Could Consent." *New York Times*, July 25.

Feinberg, Joel. 1984. *Harm to Others*. Vol. 1 of *The Moral Limits of the Criminal Law*. New York: Oxford University Press.

Feinberg, Joel, and Henry West, eds. 1977. *Moral Philosophy: Classic Texts and Contemporary Problems*. Encino, Calif.: Dickenson.

Feldman, Fred. 1992. *Confrontations with the Reaper: A Philosophical Study of the Nature and Value of Death*. New York and Oxford: Oxford University Press.

"Final Report of the Netherlands State Commission on Euthanasia: An English Summary," 1987. Trans. anon. *Bioethics* 1(2): 163–74.

Fine, Sean. 1998. "The Ethics of Death Spur Intense Debate: Who Has the Right to Let a Patient Die? The Experts Aren't Sure." *Globe and Mail*, November 14.

Fine, Sean, and David Roberts. 1998. "Life and Death: Court Decides in Wife's Favor; Judge Orders Winnipeg Hospital to Lift Do Not Resuscitate Order." *Globe and Mail*, November 14.

Fletcher, J. 1989. "The Right to Choose When to Die." *Hemlock Quarterly* (January).

Foley, K. 1991. "The Relationship of Pain and Symptom Management to Patient Requests for Physician-Assisted Suicide." *Journal of Pain and Symptom Management* 6(5): 289–97.

Foucault, Michel. 1983. "The Subject and Power." Afterword to *Michel Foucault: Beyond Structualism and Hermeneutics*. Eds. Hubert Dreyfus and Paul Rabinow. Brighton, England: Harvester Press.

———. 1988. *Michel Foucault: Politics, Philosophy, Culture: Interviews and Other Writings, 1977–1984*. Ed. Lawrence D. Kritzman. Oxford: Blackwell.

Freedman, Benjamin. 1992. "The Slippery-Slope Argument Reconstructed: Response to van der Burg." *Journal of Clinical Ethics* 3(4): 293–97.

Freud, Sigmund. 1915. "Our Attitude Towards Death." Chapter 2 of *Thoughts for the Times on War and Death. The Standard Edition of the Complete Works of Sigmund Freud*. London: Hogarth Press.

Freudenheim, Milt. 1997. "Medicare H.M.O.'s to Trim Benefits for the Elderly: Expenses Are Soaring: Cap on Government Payments Is Ending Days of Low Fees and Free Prescriptions." *New York Times*, December 22.

Fried, Charles. 1974. *Medical Experimentation: Personal Integrity and Social Policy*. Amsterdam: North Holland.

Fried, T., and M. Gillick. 1995. "The Limits of Proxy Decision Making: Over-treatment." *Cambridge Quarterly of Healthcare Ethics* 4: 524–29.

Fried, T., M. Stein, P. O'Sullivan, et al. 1993. "Limits of Patient Autonomy: Physician Attitudes and Practices Regarding Life-Sustaining Treatments and Euthanasia." *Archives of Internal Medicine* 153: 722–28.

Fulton, Robert, et al. 1976. *Death, Grief and Bereavement: A Bibliography, 1845–1975*. New York: Arno Press.

Garret, J., R. Harris, J. Norburn, D. Patrick, and M. Danis. 1993. "Life-Sustaining Treatments During Terminal Illness: Who Wants What?" *Journal of General Internal Medicine* 8: 361–68.

Garrow, David J. 1996. "The Justices' Life-or-Death Choices," *New York Times*, April 7.

———. 1997. "Letting the Public Decide About Assisted Suicide: The Court Couldn't Duck Abortion and Contraception Forever. This Moral Issue, Too, Will Be Back." *New York Times*, June 29.

Gay, Kathlyn. 1993. *The Right to Die: Public Controversy, Private Matter (Issue and Debate)*. Brookfield, Conn.: Millbrook Press.

Geis, Sally B., and Donald Messer. 1997. *How Shall We Die? Helping Christians Debate Assisted Suicide.* New York: Abingdon Press.

Gentles, Ian. 1991. "If Mercy Killing Becomes Legal," *The Globe and Mail,* November, 19, 1991.

———. 1995a. *Euthanasia and Assisted Suicide: The Current Debate.* Toronto: Stoddart.

———. 1995b. "Senate Report on Euthanasia: Pro and Con." *The Globe and Mail,* June 8.

Genuis, Stephen J., et al. 1994. "Public Attitudes Toward the Right to Die." *Canadian Medical Association Journal* 150(5): 701–708.

Gifford-Jones, W. 1995. "Northern Territory Shows Its Compassion on Euthanasia Issue." *Financial Post,* December 30.

Gilbert, Susan. 1996. "When Savings Run Out, Some Shun Lifesaving," *New York Times,* August 14.

———. 1998. "Elderly Seek Longer Life, Regardless." *New York Times,* February 10.

Gillick, M., and T. Fried. 1995. "The Limits of Proxy Decision Making: Undertreatment." *Cambridge Quarterly of Healthcare Ethics* 4: 172–77.

Gillick, M., K. Hesse, and N. Mazzapica. 1993. "Medical Technology at the End of Life: What Would Physicians and Nurses Want for Themselves?" *Archives of Internal Medicine* 153: 2542–47.

Gilligan, Carol. 1982. *In a Different Voice: Psychological Theory and Women's Development.* Cambridge and London: Harvard University Press.

Gillon, Raanan. 1992. *Philosophical Medical Ethics.* Chichester, N.Y.: John Wiley and Sons.

Glick, Shimon M. 1997. "Unlimited Human Autonomy—A Cultural Bias?" *New England Journal of Medicine* 336(13): 954–56.

Goddard, M. 1992. "Hospice Care in the Future: Economic Evaluation May Be Useful." *Cancer Topics* 9(1): 10–11.

Goldberg, Carey. 1997a. "Oregon Braces for New Right-to-Die Fight," *New York Times,* June 17.

———. 1997b. "Oregon Moves Nearer to New Vote on Allowing Assisted Suicide," *New York Times,* June 10.

Goodman, Walter. 1996. "A Husband Defends His Decision to Kill His Wife," *New York Times,* September 26.

Gorovitz, Samuel et al., eds. 1983. *Moral Problems in Medicine,* 2d ed. Englewood Cliffs, N.J.: Prentice-Hall.

Graber, Glenn, and Jennifer Chassman. 1993. "Assisted Suicide Is Not Voluntary Active Euthanasia, But It's Awfully Close." *Journal of the American Geriatrics Society* 41(1): 88–89.

Greenhouse, Linda. 1995. "Justices Decline to Hear Appeals Involving Assisted Suicide." *New York Times,* April 25.

———. 1996a. "Clinton Administration Asks Supreme Court to Rule Against

Assisted Suicide: Contrasting Life Support Withheld and Death Brought About." *New York Times*, November 13.

———. 1996b. "High Court to Say if the Dying Have a Right to Suicide Help." *New York Times*, October 2.

———. 1996c. "An Issue for a Reluctant Court." *New York Times*, October 6.

———. 1997a. "Appealing to the Law's Brooding Spirit." *New York Times*, July 6.

———. 1997b. "Assisted Suicide Clears a Hurdle in Highest Court." *New York Times*, October 15.

———. 1997c. "Benchmarks of Justice: In 9 Extraordinary Months, the High Court Developed a Vast Panorama of Landmarks." *New York Times*, July 1.

———. 1997d. "Court, 9–0, Upholds State Laws Prohibiting Assisted Suicide: No Help For Dying." *New York Times*, June 27.

———. 1997e. "High Court Hears 2 Cases Involving Assisted Suicide. Justices, in an Unusually Personal Session, Reveal Their Reluctance to Intercede." *New York Times*, January 9.

Griffiths, John. 1994. "The Regulation of Euthanasia and Related Medical Procedures that Shorten Life in the Netherlands." *Medical Law International* 1(2): 137–58.

———. 1995. "Assisted Suicide in the Netherlands: Postscript to Chabot." *Modern Law Review* 58: 895–97.

Grollman, Earl A. 1970. *Talking About Death*. Boston: Beacon Press.

Gross, Jane. 1997a. "Doctor at Center of Supreme Court Case on Assisted Suicide." *New York Times*, January 1.

———. 1997b. "Wanting a Chance to Choose Their Time: Breast Cancer Patients Say Court Overlooked Them on Assisted Suicide." *New York Times*, June 30.

Gunnell, D., and S. Frankel. 1994. "Prevention of Suicide: Aspirations and Evidence." *British Medical Journal* 308: 1227–33.

Gutmann, Stephanie. 1996. "Death and the Maiden." *New Republic* (June 24): 20–21, 24, 28.

Haberman, Clyde. 1997. "The Suicidal Still Call Out in Desperation." *New York Times*, January 31.

Hamel, Ronald, and Edwin DuBose, eds. 1996. *Must We Suffer Our Way to Death? Cultural and Theological Perspectives on Death by Choice*. Dallas: Southern Methodist University Press.

Hare, J., C. Pratt, and C. Nelson. 1992. "Agreement Between Patients and Their Self-Selected Surrogates on Difficult Medical Decisions." *Archives of Internal Medicine* 152: 1049–54.

Harman, Gilbert. 1986. *Change in View: Principles of Reasoning*. Cambridge: MIT Press.

Heap, M., R. Munglani, J. Klinck, and A. Males. 1993. "Elderly Patients' Preferences Concerning Life-Support Treatment." *Anaesthesia* 48: 1027–33.

Helme, T. 1991. "Stances Towards Euthanasia." *Psychiatric Bulletin* 15: 1–3.

Hendin, Herbert. 1996. *Seduced by Death: Doctors, Patients, and the Dutch Cure*. New York: W. W. Norton.

Hendin, Herbert, Chris Rutenfrans, and Zbigniew Zyliez. 1997. "JAMA: Another Journal Warns of Abuses in the Netherlands." *New York Times*, June 24.

Hentoff, Nat. 1996. "Front-Line Resistors Fight Kevorkian's Easy Death." *Globe and Mail*, August 24.

Herszenhorn, David M. 1997. "Writer Jailed for Assisting Wife's Suicide Reveals That He Suffocated Her." *New York Times*, June 19.

Hess, Henry. 1997a. "Doctor Faces New Charges: Hearing Delayed in Case of AIDS Patient's Suicide and Physician's Actions." *Globe and Mail*, February 4.

———. 1997b. "MD Admits Assisting Suicide: Doctor to Be Sentenced in March on Two Counts of Aiding Patients Who Wanted to Die." *Globe and Mail*, December 23.

Hiller, T., J. Patterson, M. Hodges, and M. Rosenberg. 1995. "Physicians as Patients: Choices Regarding Their Own Resuscitation." *Archives of Internal Medicine* 155: 1289–93.

Hinton, John. 1967. *Dying*. New York: Penguin.

Hoefler, James. 1994. *Culture, Medicine, Politics, and the Right to Die*. Boulder, Colo., and Oxford: Westview Press.

———. 1997. *Managing Death: The First Guide for Patients, Family Members, and Care Providers on Forgoing Treatment at the End of Life*. Boulder, Colo., and New York: Westview Press, HarperCollins.

Hofsess, John. 1992. "Killing Off the Right to Die." *Globe and Mail*, February 27.

———. 1995. "How Will the Senate Committee See Assisted Suicide?" *Globe and Mail*, May 4.

Honderich, Ted, ed. 1995. *The Oxford Companion to Philosophy*. Oxford: Oxford University Press.

Hood, Ann. 1997. "Rage Against the Dying of the Light." *New York Times*, August 2.

Hook, Sidney. 1988. "The Uses of Death." *New York Review* 25(7): 22–25.

Howard, R., and D. Miller. 1995. "The Persistent Vegetative State." *British Medical Journal* 310: 341–42.

Howe, Edmund G. 1992. "Caveats Regarding Slippery Slopes and Physicians' Moral Conscience." *Journal of Clinical Ethics* 3(4): 251–56.

Hudson, Liam. 1996. "The Age of Alzheimer's." *Medicine*, January 12.

Hume, David. [1776] 1826. "Essay on Suicide." In *The Philosophic Works of David Hume*. Edinburgh: Black and Tait.

———. [1888] 1955. *A Treatise on Human Nature*. Ed. L. A. Selby-Bigge. Oxford: Oxford University Press.

———. [1776] 1963. "My Own Life." In *Essays: Moral, Political and Literary*. Oxford: Oxford University Press.

Humphry, Derek. 1992a. *Dying with Dignity.* New York: Birch Lane Press.

———. 1992b. *Final Exit: The Practicalities of Self-Deliverance and Assisted Suicide for the Dying.* New York: Dell.

———. 1993a. "Derek Humphry Discusses Death with Dignity with Thomasine Kushner." *Cambridge Quarterly of Healthcare Ethics* 2(1): 57–61.

———. 1993b. *Lawful Exit: The Limits of Freedom for Help in Dying.* Junction City, Oreg.: Norris Lane Press.

———. 1994. "Suicide by Asphyxiation After the Publication of *Final Exit.*" *New England Journal of Medicine* 330(14): 1017.

Humphry, Derek, and A. Wickett. 1986. *The Right to Die—Understanding Euthanasia.* New York: Harper and Row. (Reprinted 1990 by the Hemlock Society, Eugene, Oreg.)

Illich, Ivan. 1976. *Limits to Medicine.* New York: Marion Boyars.

Iserson, Kenneth V. 1991. "Forgoing Prehospital Care: Should Ambulance Staff Always Resuscitate?" *Journal of Medical Ethics* 17: 19–24.

Jacobson, Stanley. 1995. "Depression as a Healthy Response." *Globe and Mail,* June 10.

James, William. 1897. "The Will to Believe." In *The Will to Believe and Other Essays in Popular Philosophy.* New York: Longman's Green.

Jamison, Stephen. 1996. *Final Acts of Love: Families, Friends, and Assisted Dying.* New York: Putnam Publishing Group.

Jarvik, Lissy. 1979. *Psychological Symptoms and Cognitive Loss in the Elderly.* New York: Halsted.

Jecker, N., and L. Schneiderman. 1993. "Medical Futility: The Duty Not to Treat." *Cambridge Quarterly of Healthcare Ethics* 2: 151–59.

———. 1994. "Is Dying Young Worse than Dying Old?" *Gerontologist* 34(1): 66–72.

Jeffrey, D. 1994. "Active Euthanasia—Time for a Decision." *British Journal of General Practice* (March): 136–38.

———. 1996. "Saying Goodbye in a Good Way: Observations on Palliative Care in the Netherlands." *Proceedings of the Royal College of Physicians* (Edinburgh) 26: 216–23.

Jochemsen, H. 1994. "Euthanasia in Holland: An Ethical Critique of the New Law." *Journal of Medical Ethics* 20: 212–17.

Johnson, Dirk. 1997. "Nurse with Tender Touch Is Held in 6 Killings." *New York Times,* December 31.

Johnson, Linda A. 1997. "Kevorkian Aids N.J. Woman: MS Patient Ends Life in Mich." *Times* (Trenton, N.J., *via* Associated Press), July 3.

Johnston, Brian. 1994. *Death as a Salesman: What's Wrong with Assisted Suicide.* Sacramento: New Regency Publishing.

Judis, John B. 1997. "Careless: A Poison Pill for Medicare." *New Republic,* July 28.

Kamisar, Yale. 1991. "Euthanasia Legislation: Some Nonreligious Objections." In *Biomedical Ethics.* 3d ed. Eds. Thomas A. Mappes and Jane S. Zembaty. New York: McGraw-Hill.

―――. 1993. "Are Laws Against Assisted Suicide Unconstitutional?" *Hastings Center Report* 23(3): 32–41.

―――. 1998. "Details Doom Assisted-Suicide Measures: Moving Stories vs. Legislative Reality." *New York Times*, November 4.

Kane, Francis I. 1985. "Keeping Elizabeth Bouvia Alive for the Public Good." *Hastings Center Report* 15(6): 5–9.

Kant, Immanuel. "Suicide." In *Biomedical Ethics*. 3d ed. Eds. Thomas A. Mappes and Jane S. Zembaty. New York: McGraw-Hill.

Kass, L. 1993. "Is There a Right to Die?" *Hastings Center Report* (January–February): 34–43.

Kastenbaum, Robert J. 1964. *New Thoughts on Old Age*. New York: Springer.

―――. 1967. "Suicide as the Preferred Way of Death." In *Suicidology: Contemporary Developments*. Ed. Edwin Shneidman. New York: Grune and Stratton.

―――. 1991. *Death, Society, and Human Experience*. New York: Merrill.

―――. 1992. *The Psychology of Death*. New York: Springer.

Kastenbaum, Robert, and Beatrice Kastenbaum, eds. 1989. *Encyclopedia of Death*. Phoenix: Oryx Press.

Kaufmann, Walter, ed. 1954. *The Portable Nietzsche*. New York: Viking Press.

Kaveny, M. Cathleen, and John P. Langan. 1996. "The Doctor's Call." *New York Times*, July 15.

Kearl, Michael C. 1989. *Endings: A Sociology of Death and Dying*. New York: Oxford University Press.

Keizer, Bert. 1997. *Dancing with Mister D: Notes on Life and Death*. New York: Doubleday.

Kellogg, F., M. Crain, J. Corwin, and P. Brickner. 1992. "Life-Sustaining Interventions in Frail Elderly Persons—Talking About Choices." *Archives of Internal Medicine* 152: 2317–20.

Kennedy, I., and A. Grubb. 1994. *Medical Law, Text With Materials*, 2d ed. London: Butterworth.

Kennedy, Randy. 1998. "Doctor Is Arraigned in Assisted Suicide: Veterinarian Is Said to Admit Role in Terminally Ill Friend's Death." *New York Times*, October 15.

Kevles, Daniel J. 1995. "We All Must Die; Who Can Tell Us When?" *New York Times Book Review*, May 7.

Kielstein, R., and H. Sass. 1993. "Using Stories to Assess Values and Establish Medical Directives." *Kennedy Institute of Ethics Journal* 3(3): 303–25.

Kilborn, Peter T. 1998. "Largest H.M.O.'s Cutting the Poor and the Elderly: A Managed-Care Retreat: Insurers Cite Losses and Low Government Payments in Medicaid and Medicare." *New York Times*, July 6.

Kimsma, G., and E. Leeuwen. 1993. "Dutch Euthanasia: Background, Practice, and Present Justifications." *Cambridge Quarterly of Healthcare Ethics* 2: 19–35.

Kluge, Eike-Henner. 1975. *The Practice of Death*. New Haven, Conn.: Yale University Press.

Knight, Ben. 1996. "Death with Dignity: Our Last Right." In *Readers Showcase*. Toronto: Coles/Smithbooks.

Kolata, Gina. 1996a. "1 in 5 Nurses Tell Survey They Helped Patients Die." *New York Times*, May 23.

———. 1996b. "In Shift, Prospects for Survival Will Decide Liver Transplants." *New York Times*, November 15.

———. 1997a. "Alzheimer Patients Present a Lesson on Human Dignity." *New York Times*, January 1.

———. 1997b. "Ethicists Struggle Against the Tyranny of the Anecdote." *New York Times*, June 24.

———. 1997c. "Group Proposes a New System on Liver Transplant Priorities." *New York Times*, June 27.

———. 1997d. "Living Wills Aside, Dying Cling to Hope." *New York Times*, January 15.

———. 1997e. " 'Passive Euthanasia' in Hospitals Is the Norm, Doctors Say." *New York Times*, June 28.

———. 1997f. "When Morphine Fails to Kill." *New York Times*, July 23.

Komesaroff, P., J. Lickiss, M. Parker, and M. Ashby. 1995. "The Euthanasia Controversy: Decision-Making In Extreme Cases." *Medical Journal of Australia* 162: 594–97.

Kottow, M. H. 1988. "Euthanasia After the Holocaust—Is It Possible?: A Report from the Federal Republic of Germany." *Bioethics* 2(1): 58–69.

Krausz, Michael, ed. 1989. *Relativism: Interpretation and Confrontation*. Notre Dame: University of Notre Dame Press.

Kristof, Nicholas. 1997. "Japanese Parents Wonder Who Will Look After Them: As the Baby-Boom Generation Approaches Retirement, Untraditional Children Are No Longer Sharing Their Homes and Caring for Older Family Members." *Globe and Mail*, August 14.

Kristol, Elizabeth. 1993. "Soothing Moral Shroud." *Washington Post*, December 3.

Krynski, M., A. Tymchuk, and J. Ouslander. 1994. "How Informed Can Consent Be? New Light on Comprehension Among Elderly People Making Decisions About Enteral Tube Feeding." *Gerontologist* 34(1): 36–43.

Kübler-Ross, Elisabeth. 1969. *On Death and Dying*. New York: Macmillan.

Kuhse, Helga. 1986. *Willing to Listen, Wanting to Die*. Ringwood, Victoria: Penguin Books.

———. 1997. *Caring: Nurses, Women, and Ethics*. Oxford: Blackwell.

Kung, Hans, and Walter Jens. 1995. *Dying with Dignity: A Plea for Personal Responsibility*. New York: Continuum.

Kushner, Howard. 1989. *Self-Destruction in the Promised Land*. New Brunswick, N.J.: Rutgers University Press.

Kutner, L. 1969. "Due Process of Euthanasia: The Living Will, a Proposal." *Indiana Law Journal* 539: 539–54.

Ladd, John, ed. 1979. *Ethical Issues Relating to Life and Death*. New York: Oxford University Press.

Lambert, P., J. Gibson, and P. Nathanson. 1990. "The Values History: An Innovation in Surrogate Medical Decision-Making." *Law, Medicine and Health Care* 18(3): 202–12.

Latimer, E. 1991. "Ethical Decision-Making in the Care of the Dying and Its Applications to Clinical Practice." *Journal of Pain and Symptom Management* 6(5): 329–36.

Laurence, Margaret. 1964. *The Stone Angel*. Toronto: McClelland and Stewart.

Law Reform Commission of Canada. 1982. *Euthanasia, Aiding Suicide and Cessation of Treatment*. Working Paper 28.

Leary, Warren E. 1997. "Not Enough Is Done to Ease End of Life, Panel Says." *New York Times*, June 5.

Lee, M., and L. Ganzini. 1994. "The Effect of Recovery from Depression on Preferences for Life-Sustaining Therapy in Older Patients." *Journal of Gerontology* 49(1): M15-M21.

Leonard-Taitz, J. 1992. "Euthanasia, the Right to Die and the Law in South Africa." *Medicine and Law* 11: 597–610.

Lessenberry, Jack. 1996a. "Kevorkian Indicted on Charges of Helping in Three Suicides." *New York Times*, November 1.

———. 1996b. "Kevorkian Is Arrested and Charged in a Suicide." *New York Times*, November 7.

———. 1996c. "Prosecutor Goes Against Tide, Going After Kevorkian." *New York Times*, November 25.

———. 1996d. "Many Turning to Internet for Aid with Suicide." *New York Times*, July 15.

———. 1996e. "Specialist Testifies Depression Was Issue in Kevorkian Cases." *New York Times*, April 23.

Levin, Jack, and William Levin. 1980. *Ageism: Prejudice and Discrimination against the Elderly*. Belmont, Calif.: Wadsworth.

Levin, Martin. 1996. "Verdicts on Verdicts About Easeful Death." *Globe and Mail*, August 10.

Lewin, Tamar. 1997. "New Guidelines on Sexual Harassment Tell Schools When a Kiss Is Just a Peck." *New York Times*, March 15.

Lewis, Neil A. 1998. "2 with Intimate Knowledge of How to Look at Death." *New York Times*, June 27.

Lifton, Robert Jay. 1987. *The Future of Immortality and Other Essays for a Nuclear Age*. New York: Basic Books.

Lockwood, Michael, ed. 1985. *Moral Dilemmas in Modern Medicine*. Oxford: Oxford University Press.

Loewy, E. H. 1992. "Advance Directives and Surrogate Laws—Ethical Instruments or Moral Cop-Out?" *Archives of Internal Medicine* 152: 1973–76.

———. 1995. "Compassion, Reason, and Moral Judgement." *Cambridge Quarterly of Healthcare Ethics* 4(4): 466–75.

Logue, Barbara. 1993. *Last Rights: Death Control and the Elderly in America.* Oxford: Maxwell Macmillan.

Longo, Dianne C., and Reg Arthur Williams. 1986. *Clinical Practice in Psychosocial Nursing: Assessment and Intervention.* Norwalk, Conn.: Appleton-Century-Crofts.

Lown, Bernard. 1997. *The Lost Art of Healing.* New York: Houghton Mifflin.

Lowy, C. 1988. "The Doctrine of Substituted Judgment in Medical Decision Making." *Bioethics* 2(1): 15–21.

Lynn, Joanne, ed. 1986, *By No Extraordinary Means: The Choice to Forgo Life-Sustaining Food and Water.* Bloomington and Indianapolis: Indiana University Press.

Lynn, Joanne, and James Childress. 1986. "Must Patients Always Be Given Food and Water: Is It Killing?" In *By No Extraordinary Means.* Ed. Joanne Lynn. Bloomington and Indianapolis: Indiana University Press.

Lynn, Joanne, and J. Teno. 1993. "After the Patient Self-Determination Act—The Need for Empirical Research on Formal Advance Directives." *Hastings Center Report* (January–February): 20–24.

Maas, P., J. Delden and L. Pijnenborg. 1992. "Euthanasia and Other Medical Decisions Concerning the End of Life—An Investigation Performed Upon the Request of the Commission of Inquiry into the Medical Practice Concerning Euthanasia." *Health Policy* (Special Issue) 22(1 and 2).

Maas, P., J. Delden, L. Pijnenborg, and C. Looman. 1991. "Euthanasia and Other Medical Decisions Concerning the End of Life." *Lancet* 338: 669–74.

Makin, Kirk. 1997. "Exemptions Rarely Needed, Experts Say: Mandatory Sentences Disappearing as Judges Given Penalty Latitude for Most Crimes." *Globe and Mail*, December 2.

Malcolm, Andrew. 1990. "What Medical Science Can't Seem to Learn: When to Call It Quits." *New York Times*, December 23.

Maltsberger, John, and Mark Goldblatt, eds. 1996. *Essential Papers on Suicide.* New York: New York University Press.

Mappes, Thomas A., and Jane S. Zembaty. 1991. *Biomedical Ethics*, 3d ed. New York: McGraw-Hill.

Marcus, Eric. 1996. *Why Suicide: Answers to 200 of the Most Frequently Asked Questions About Suicide, Attempted Suicide, and Assisted Suicide.* San Francisco: Harper.

Margulies, Alfred. 1989. *The Empathic Imagination.* New York: W. W. Norton.

Markoff, John. 1990. "Programmed for Life and Death." *New York Times.* August 26.

Marshall, Andrew. 1994. "A Nasty Piece of Work: Wataru Tsurumi's Suicide Manual Makes a Killing." *Intersect*, May.

Martin, Douglas. 1989. "Creating Beauty Out of Suffering as Life Fades." *New York Times*, February 18.

Martin, R. M. 1980. "Suicide and Self-Sacrifice," in *Suicide: The Philosophical*

Issues. Eds. Margaret Pabst Battin and D. J. Mayo. New York: St. Martin's Press.

Martyn, S. R. 1994. "Substituted Judgement, Best Interests, and the Need for Best Respect." *Cambridge Quarterly of Healthcare Ethics* 3(2): 195–208.

May, William F. 1996. *Testing the Medical Covenant: Active Euthanasia and Health Care Reform.* Grand Rapids, Mich.: Eerdmans.

McDougall, Burnley. 1994. "Challenging the Oath of Hippocrates." *Globe and Mail,* March 8.

McGough, P. 1993. "Washington State Initiative 119: The First Public Vote on Legalizing Physician Assisted Death." *Cambridge Quarterly of Healthcare Ethics* 2: 63–67.

McIlroy, Anne. 1998. " 'Who Are We to Decide?' M.P. Asks of Euthanasia: Debate on Private Member's Motion Gets Personal for Some." *Globe and Mail,* February 3.

McIntosh, John L., and Nancy J. Osgood. 1986. *Suicide and the Elderly.* Westport: Greenwood Press.

McKee, Patrick. 1988. "The Aging Mind: View from Philosophy and Psychology." *Gerontologist* 28(1): 132–33.

McLean, Sheila A. M. 1989. *A Patient's Right to Know—Information Disclosure, the Doctor and the Law.* Hants, England: Aldershot; Brookfield, Vt.: Dartmouth.

———. 1993. "Letting Die or Assisting Death: How Should the Law Respond to the Patient in Persistent Vegetative State?" *Law and Medicine* (Special Issue) 11(2): 3–16.

———. 1994. "Human Rights and the Patient in a Persistent Vegetative State." *International Legal Practitioner* 19(1): 19–20.

———, ed. 1996a. *Contemporary Issues in Law, Ethics and Medicine.* Brookfield, Vt.: Dartmouth Publishing Co.

———. 1996b. *Death, Dying and the Law.* Brookfield, Vt.: Dartmouth Publishing Co.

McNulty, C. 1995. "Mentally Incapacitated Adults and Decision-Making: a Psychological Perspective—Comments on Law Commission Consultation Papers, Numbers 128, 129 and 130." *Medicine, Science and the Law* 35(2): 159–64.

Meier, D., and C. Cassel. 1983. "Euthanasia in Old Age—A Case Study and Ethical Analysis." *Journal of the American Geriatrics Society* 31(5): 294–98.

Meier, Diane E. 1998. "A Change of Heart on Assisted Suicide." *New York Times,* April 24.

Menninger, Karl. 1966. *Man Against Himself.* New York: Harvest/HBJ.

Mezey, M., L. Evans, Z. Golub, E. Murphy, and G. White. 1994. "The Patient Self-Determination Act: Sources of Concern for Nurses." *Nursing Outlook* 42(1): 30–38.

Mezey, M., and B. Latimer. 1993. "The Patient Self-Determination Act—An

Early Look at Implementation." *Hastings Center Report* (January/February): 16–20.

Mickleburgh, Rod. 1991. "Euthanasia Backed in Report," *Globe and Mail*, November 13.

Miles, S., and A. August. 1990. "Courts, Gender and the 'Right to Die.' " *Law, Medicine and Health Care* 18: 85–95.

Miller, Phillip. 1987. "Death with Dignity and the Right to Die: Sometimes Doctors Have a Duty to Hasten Death." *Journal of Medical Ethics* 13: 81–85.

Miller, R. J. 1992. "Hospice Care as an Alternative to Euthanasia." *Law Medicine and Health Care* 20(1–2): 127–32.

Mitford, Jessica. 1963. *The American Way of Death*. New York: Simon and Schuster.

Miyaji, N. T. 1993. "The Power of Compassion: Truth-Telling Among American Doctors in the Care of Dying Patients." *Social Science Medicine* 36(3): 249–64.

Molloy, D., C. Harrison, M. Farrugia, and A. Cunje. 1993. "The Canadian Experience with Advance Treatment Directives." *Humane Medicine* 9(1): 70–76.

Molotsky, Irvin. 1998. "Wife Wins Right-to-Die Case; Then a Governor Challenges It." *New York Times*, October 2.

Montaigne, Michel de. 1995. *Essays*, Bk. 2, Chap. 3, "A Custom of the Isle of Cea." Trans. John Florio. Quoted in *The Columbia Dictionary of Quotations*, 1995. New York: Columbia University Press, Microsoft *Bookshelf*, 1996–97 CD-ROM edition.

More, Ellen Singer, and Maureen A. Milligan, eds. 1994. *The Empathic Practitioner: Empathy, Gender, and Medicine*. New Brunswick, N.J.: Rutgers University Press.

Moreno, Jonathan D. 1995a. *Deciding Together: Bioethics and Moral Consensus*. New York: Oxford University Press.

———, ed. 1995b. *Arguing Euthanasia: The Controversy over Mercy Killing, Assisted Suicide, and the "Right to Die."* New York: Simon and Schuster.

Morgentaler, Henry. 1982. *Abortion and Contraception*. New York: Beaufort Books.

Mullens, Anne. 1996. *Timely Death: Considering Our Last Rights*. New York: Alfred A. Knopf.

Munson, Ronald. 1988. *Intervention and Reflection: Basic Issues in Medical Ethics*, 3d ed. Belmont, Calif.: Wadsworth.

Mydans, Seth. 1997. "Assisted Suicide: Australia Faces a Grim Reality." *New York Times*, February 2.

Nadelson, Carol C. 1993. "Ethics, Empathy and Gender in Health Care." *American Journal of Psychiatry* 150: 1309–14.

Narveson, Jan. 1986. "Moral Philosophy and Suicide." *Canadian Journal of Psychiatry* 31: 104–107.

———. 1993. *Moral Matters*. Peterborough, Ontario: Broadview Press.

Navarro, Mireya. 1997. "Assisted Suicide Decision Looms in Florida," *New York Times*, July 3.

Niebuhr, Gustav. 1996. "Dying Cardinal Lobbies Against Suicide Aid," *New York Times*, November 13.

———. 1997. "On the Furthest Fringes of Millennialism." *New York Times*, March 28.

Nietzsche, Friedrich. 1954. *Thus Spake Zarathustra* (Part One, 1883). In *The Portable Nietzsche*. Ed. Walter Kaufmann. New York: Viking Press, 1954.

Nuland, Sherwin B. 1994. *How We Die: Reflections on Life's Final Chapter*. New York: Alfred A. Knopf.

———. 1997. "How We Die Is Our Business," *New York Times*, January 13.

Oates, Joyce Carol. 1980. "The Art of Suicide." In *Suicide: The Philosophical Issues*. Eds. Margaret Pabst Battin and D. J. Mayo. New York: St. Martin's Press.

Ogden, R. 1994. *Euthanasia, Assisted Suicide and AIDS*. British Columbia: Perreault Goedman.

Ogilvie, A., and S. Potts. 1994. "Assisted Suicide for Depression: The Slippery Slope in Action?" *British Medical Journal* 309: 492–93.

Orentlicher, David. 1990. "Advance Medical Directives." *Journal of the American Medical Association* 263(17): 2365–67.

Ouslander, J., A. Tymchuk, and B. Rahbar. 1989. "Health Care Decisions Among Elderly Long-Term Care Residents and Their Potential Proxies." *Archives of Internal Medicine* 149: 1367–72.

Outhit, Jeff. 1997. "Homes May Refuse Frailest Seniors: Sickest Seniors in Middle of Funding Dispute," *The Kingston Whig-Standard*, February 13.

Ozar, David. 1992. "The Characteristics of a Valid 'Empirical' Slippery Slope Argument." *Journal of Clinical Ethics* 3(4): 301–302.

Pace, N., and S. McLean, eds. 1996. *Ethics and the Law in Intensive Care*. Oxford: Oxford University Press.

Pear, Robert. 1996. "Managed Care Officials Agree to Mastectomy Hospital Stays: Health Plans Act to Head off Federal Regulations," *New York Times*, November 15.

———. 1997. "H.M.O.'s Limiting Medicare Appeals, U.S. Inquiry Finds: Government Is Told by Court to Clarify Its Guidelines on Elderly Patients' Rights," *New York Times*, March 18.

Pearlman, Robert A., et al. 1992. "Spousal Understanding of Patient Quality of Life: Implications for Surrogate Decisions." *Journal of Clinical Ethics* 3(2): 114–21.

Pellegrino, Edmund D. 1992. "Doctors Must Not Kill." *Journal of Clinical Ethics* 3(2): 95–103.

———. 1993. "Compassion Needs Reason Too." *Journal of the American Medical Association* 270(7): 874–75.

Pence, G. E. 1995. *Classic Cases in Medical Ethics*, 2d ed. New York: McGraw-Hill.

Perlin, Seymour, ed. 1975. *A Handbook for the Study of Suicide.* Oxford: Oxford University Press.

Pijnenborg, L., et al. 1995. "Withdrawal or Withholding of Treatment at the End of Life—Results of a Nationwide Study." *Archives of Internal Medicine* 155: 286–92.

Pohier, Jacques, and Dietmar Mieth. 1985. *Suicide and the Right to Die.* Edinburgh: T. and T. Clark.

Powell, Tia, and Donald B. Kornfeld. 1993. "On Promoting Rational Treatment, Not Rational Suicide." *Journal of Clinical Ethics* 4(4): 334–35.

Prado, C. G. 1984. *Making Believe: Philosophical Reflections on Fiction.* Westport, Conn.: Greenwood Group.

———. 1986. *Rethinking How We Age: A New View of the Aging Mind.* New York and Westport, Conn.: Greenwood Group.

———. 1990. *The Last Choice: Preemptive Suicide in Advanced Age.* New York and Westport, Conn.: Greenwood Group.

———. 1995. *Starting with Foucault: An Introduction to Genealogy.* Boulder, Colo., and San Francisco: Westview Press, HarperCollins.

———. 1998. *The Last Choice: Preemptive Suicide in Advanced Age,* 2d ed. New York and Westport, Conn.: Greenwood and Praeger Presses.

President's Commission for the Study of Ethical Problems in Medicine and Biomedical and Behavioral Research. 1983. *Deciding to Forego Life-Sustaining Treatment—A Report on the Ethical, Medical, and Legal Issues in Treatment Decisions.* New York: Concern for Dying.

Purdum, Todd. 1997. "Tapes Left by 39 in Cult Suicide Suggest Comet Was Sign to Die." *New York Times,* March 28.

Quill, Timothy. 1991. "Death and Dignity—A Case of Individualized Decision Making." *New England Journal of Medicine* 324(10): 691–94.

———. 1993a. *Death and Dignity: Making Choices and Taking Charge.* New York: W. W. Norton.

———. 1993b. "Doctor, I Want to Die. Will You Help Me?" *Journal of the American Medical Association* 270(7): 870–73.

———. 1995. "You Promised Me I Wouldn't Die Like This!—A Bad Death as a Medical Emergency." *Archives of Internal Medicine* 155: 1250–54.

———. 1996. *A Midwife Through the Dying Process: Stories of Healing and Hard Choices at the End of Life.* Baltimore: Johns Hopkins University Press.

Quill, T., C. Cassel, and D. Meier. 1992. "Care of the Hopelessly Ill—Proposed Clinical Criteria for Physician Assisted Suicide." *New England Journal of Medicine* 327(19): 1380–84.

Quill, Timothy, and Betty Rollin. 1996. "Dr. Kevorkian Runs Wild," *New York Times,* August 29.

Rabinovitz, Jonathan. 1997. "Suicide Brings to Life a Legal Quandary: Ambiguities in Case of a Man Charged with Helping His Wife to Die." *New York Times,* July 8.

Rachels, James. 1986. *The End of Life: Euthanasia and Morality.* Oxford: Oxford University Press.

Regan, Tom, ed. 1980. *Matters of Life and Death.* Philadelphia: Temple University Press.

Reichenbach, B. 1987. "Euthanasia and the Active-Passive Distinction." *Bioethics* 1(1): 51–73.

Reilly B., R. Magnussen, J. Ross, et al. 1994. "Can We Talk? Inpatient Discussions About Advance Directives in a Community Hospital." *Archives of Internal Medicine* 154: 2299–2308.

Reno, J. 1992. "A Little Help from My Friends: The Legal Status of Assisted Suicide." *Creighton Law Review* 25: 1151–83.

Reyk, P. 1994. *Choosing to Die—A Booklet for People Thinking about Euthanasia and for Those Asked to Assist.* Sydney: AIDS Council of New South Wales.

Roberts, David. 1997. "Latimer Receives 1 Year in Jail: Judge Waives Life Sentence." *Globe and Mail,* December 2.

Robertson, J. Cruzan. 1990. "No Rights Violated." *Hastings Center Report* (September/October): 8–9.

———. 1991. "Second Thoughts on Living Wills." *Hastings Center Report* (November/December): 6–9.

Robinson, Paul. 1984. *Criminal Law Defenses.* St. Paul, Minn.: West.

Robinson, Wade L., and Michael S. Pritchard, eds. 1979. *Medical Responsibility.* Clifton, N.J.: Humana Press.

Rodriguez, G. 1990. "An Opposing View. Routine Discussion of Advance Health Care Directives: Are We Ready?" *Journal of Family Practice* 31(6): 656–59.

Roe, J., M. Goldstein, K. Massey, and D. Pascoe. 1992. "Durable Power of Attorney for Health Care: A Survey of Senior Center Participants." *Archives of Internal Medicine* 152: 292–96.

Rorty, Richard. 1982. *The Consequences of Pragmatism.* Minneapolis: University of Minnesota Press.

———. 1989. *Contingency, Irony, and Solidarity.* Cambridge: Cambridge University Press.

———. 1992. "A Pragmatist View of Rationality and Cultural Difference." *Philosophy East and West* 42(4): 581–96.

Rosen, Jeffrey. 1996. "What Right to Die?" *New Republic* (June 24): 28–31.

———. 1997. "Nine Votes for Judicial Restraint: The Court Rejects a 'Right to Die'—and the Legacy of *Roe* v. *Wade.*" *New York Times,* June 29.

Rosenberg, Charles E. 1996. "Seduced by Death," *New York Times Book Review,* November 24.

Rosenthal, Elizabeth. 1997. "When a Healer Is Asked, 'Help Me Die.'" *New York Times,* March 13.

Ross, Oakland. 1991. "The Right to Die: Going Gently," *Globe and Mail,* September 14.

Roy, David J., John R. Williams, and Bernard M. Dickens. 1994. *Bioethics in Canada*. Scarborough, Ontario: Prentice-Hall, Canada.

Sabatino, Charles. 1993. "Surely the Wizard Will Help Us, Toto? Implementing the Patient Self-Determination Act." *Hastings Center Report* (January/February): 12–16.

Sacks M., and I. Kemperman. 1992. "*Final Exit* as a Manual for Suicide in Depressed Patients." *American Journal of Psychiatry* 149(6): 842.

Salmon, Phillida. 1985. *Living in Time*. London: J. M. Dent and Sons.

Samuels, A. 1996. "The Advance Directive (or Living Will)." *Medicine, Science and the Law*, 36(1):2–8.

Sandel, Michael. 1997. "The Hard Questions: Last Rights." *New Republic* (April 14): 27.

Sanders, Stephanie. 1992. "A Time to Live or a Time to Die?" *Nursing Times* 88(45): 34–36.

Saultz, J. 1990. "An Affirmative View. Routine Discussion of Advance Health Care Directives: Are We Ready?" *Journal of Family Practice* 31(6): 653–56.

Saunders, John. 1997. "Nurse Present at Scores of Assisted Suicide Deaths: Making Aided Suicide Legal Would Ensure 'Proper Consultation,' Activist Says." *Globe and Mail*, December 23.

———. 1998. "A Time to Die: Medical Cases Such as That Involving Dr. Nancy Morrison Stir Strong Feelings in People Who Wish a Dying Friend or Relative Had Been Kept Alive Longer—or Let Go Sooner. How Do We Determine the Line between Relieving Pain and Hastening Death?" *Globe and Mail*, March 7.

Savulescu, Julian. 1994a. "Rational Desires and the Limitation of Life-Sustaining Treatment." *Bioethics* 8(3): 191–222.

———. 1994b. "Treatment Limitation Decisions Under Uncertainty: The Value of Subsequent Euthanasia." *Bioethics* 8(1): 49–73.

Sawyer, D.M. 1994. "What Do Canadian MDs Think About Euthanasia? An Update Following the CMA Annual Meeting," *Canadian Medical Association Journal* 150(3): 395–98.

Schafer, Arthur. 1990. "Treading the Finest of Lines," *Globe and Mail*, August 16.

Schaffner, K. F. 1988. "Recognizing the Tragic Choice: Food, Water, and the Right to Assisted Suicide." *Critical Care Medicine* 16(10): 1063–68.

Scheper, T., and S. Duursma. 1994. "Euthanasia: The Dutch Experience." *Age and Aging* 23: 3–8.

Schneiderman, Lawrence, and J. Arras. 1985. "Counseling Patients to Counsel Physicians on Future Health Care in the Event of Patient Incompetence." *Annals of Internal Medicine* 102: 693–98.

Schneiderman, Lawrence, R. Pearlman, R. Kaplan, J. Anderson, and E. Rosenberg. 1992. "Relationship of General Advance Directive Instructions To Specific Life-Sustaining Treatment Preferences in Patients with Serious Illness." *Archives of Internal Medicine* 152: 2114–22.

Schneiderman, Lawrence, et al. 1993. "Do Physicians' Own Preferences for Life-Sustaining Treatment Influence Their Perceptions of Patients' Preferences?" *Journal of Clinical Ethics* 4(1): 28–33.

Scott, Janny. 1997. "An Issue That Won't Die: Court's Ruling on Doctor-Assisted Suicide Leaves Some Basic Questions Unresolved." *New York Times*, June 27.

Seckler, A., D. Meier, M. Mulvihill, et al. 1991. "Substituted Judgment: How Accurate Are Proxy Predictions?" *Annals of Internal Medicine* 115(2): 92–98.

Sedler, Robert. 1993. "The Constitution and Hastening Inevitable Death." *Hastings Center Report*, 23(5):20–25.

Self, Thomas W. 1998. "One Man's Battle with the Managed-Care Monster." *New York Times*, July 13.

Selzer, Richard. 1994. *Raising the Dead*. New York: Whittle/Viking.

Senate of Canada. 1995. *Of Life and Death: Report of the Special Senate Committee on Euthanasia and Assisted Suicide*. June.

Seneca. 1969. *Letters from a Stoic*. Letter 77. Trans. Robin Campbell. Baltimore: Penguin Books.

Shapiro, R. 1992. "Unanswered Questions Surrounding the Patient Self-Determination Act." *Cambridge Quarterly of Healthcare Ethics* 2: 117–19.

Shapiro, R., A. Derse, M. Gottlieb, D. Schiedermayer, and M. Olson. 1994. "Willingness to Perform Euthanasia: A Survey of Physician Attitudes." *Archives of Internal Medicine* 154: 575–84.

Shavelson, Lonny. 1995. *A Chosen Death: The Dying Confront Assisted Suicide*. New York: Simon and Schuster.

Shenon, Philip. 1995. "Australian Euthanasia Legislation Sparks Mixture of Relief, Rage." *Globe and Mail*, July 29.

Sherstobitoff, Nicholas. 1995. "Is Robert Latimer's Life Sentence 'Cruel and Unusual Punishment'? The Sentence Should Stand." *Globe and Mail*, July 20.

Shipp, E. R. 1988. "New York's Highest Court Rejects Family's Plea in Right-to-Die Case" (and transcript excerpts) and "Many Courts Have Upheld Right to Die." *New York Times*, October 15.

Shneidman, Edwin. 1984. *Death: Current Perspectives*, 3d ed. Mountain View, Calif.: Mayfield.

———. 1993. *Suicide as Psychache: A Clinical Approach to Self-Destructive Behavior*. Northvale, N.J.: Aronson.

———. 1996. *The Suicidal Mind*. New York: Oxford University Press.

Shneidman, Edwin, ed. 1969. *On the Nature of Suicide*. San Francisco: Jossey-Bass.

———. 1976. *Suicidology: Contemporary Developments*. New York: Grune and Stratton.

Shuchman, Dr. Miriam. 1998. "Second Opinion: Patient's Beloved Deserve a Say." *Globe and Mail*, November 17.

Simpson, Michael A. 1979. *The Facts of Death*. Englewood Cliffs, N.J.: Spectrum/Prentice-Hall.

――――. 1987. *Dying, Death, and Grief: A Critical Bibliography*. Pittsburgh: University of Pittsburgh Press.

Singer, Peter. 1979. *Practical Ethics*. Cambridge: Cambridge University Press.

Skegg, P. 1984. *Law, Ethics and Medicine—Studies in Medical Law*. Oxford: Clarendon Press.

Smith, G. II. 1993. "Reviving the Swan, Extending the Curse of Methuselah, or Adhering to the Kevorkian Ethic?" *Cambridge Quarterly of Healthcare Ethics*, 2: 49–56.

Smith, Wesley. 1997. *Forced Exit: The Slippery Slope from Assisted Suicide to Legalized Murder*. New York: Times Books.

Sobel, Dava. 1991. "They Rarely Leave a Note." *New York Times Book Review*, April 14.

Sommerville, Ann. 1995. "Remembrance of Conversations Past: Oral Advance Statements About Medical Treatment." *British Medical Journal* 310: 1663–65.

Southard, Samuel. 1991. *Death and Dying: A Bibliographical Survey*. New York: Greenwood Press.

Spicker, Stuart, Stanley Ingman, and Ian Lawson, eds. 1987. *Ethical Dimensions of Geriatric Care: Value Conflicts for the 21st Century*. Dordrecht: Reidel.

Spiro, Howard, Mary G. McCrea Curnen, Enid Peschel, and Deborah St. James, eds. 1994. *Empathy and the Practice of Medicine: Beyond Pills and the Scalpel*. New Haven, Conn., and London: Yale University Press.

Stanley, Joel, ed. 1992. "The Appleton International Conference: Developing Guidelines for Decisions to Forgo Life-Prolonging Treatment." *Journal of Medical Ethics* 18 (Supplement): 1–22.

Steinfels, Peter. 1997a. "Beliefs: The Issue of Doctor-Assisted Suicide Is Put on the Scales of Justice, and Philosophers Weigh In." *New York Times*, April 5.

――――. 1997b. "Beliefs: The Justices of the Supreme Court, Preparing Landmark Opinions, Are Now Writing about Doctor-Assisted Suicide. They're Hardly Alone." *New York Times*, June 14.

――――. 1997c. "Perspective: Doctor-Assisted Suicide." *New York Times*, January 11.

――――. 1998a. "Beliefs: A Longtime Leader in Biomedical Ethics Reflects on His Field's Explosive Growth, the Backlash against It and 'False Hopes' in America's Health Care Quest." *New York Times*, May 2.

――――. 1998b. "Beliefs: Doctor-Assisted Suicide in Oregon: An Idea that Complicates Health Care for the Poor and Challenges Government Neutrality." *New York Times*, March 7.

Steinfels, Peter, and R.M. Veatch, eds. 1975. *Death Inside Out*. New York: Harper and Row.

Steinhauer, Jennifer. 1998. "Was It Mercy or Murder? Veterinarian's Arrest Puts

Focus on Pacts to Help the Terminally Ill Commit Suicide." *New York Times*, October 17.

Stelter, K., B. Elliott, and C. Bruno. 1992. "Living Will Completion in Older Adults." *Archives of Internal Medicine* 152: 954–59.

Stevens, C., and R. Hassan. 1994. "Management of Death, Dying and Euthanasia: Attitudes and Practices of Medical Practitioners in South Australia." *Journal of Medical Ethics* 20: 41–46.

Stevens, M. L. Tina. 1997. "What *Quinlan* Can Tell Kevorkian About the Right to Die." *Humanist* 57(2): 10–14.

Stillion, Judith M. 1989. *Suicide Across the Life Span—Premature Exits*. New York: Hemisphere.

Stolberg, Sheryl Gay. 1997a. "Considering the Unthinkable: Protocol for Assisted Suicide." *New York Times*, June 11.

———. 1997b. "Cries of the Dying Awaken Doctors to a New Approach, Palliative Care." *New York Times*, June 30.

———. 1997c. "The Good Death: Embracing a Right to Die Well." *New York Times*, June 29.

———. 1998a. "As Life Ebbs, So Does Time to Elect Comforts of Hospice." *New York Times*, March 4.

———. 1998b. "Assisted Suicides Are Rare, Survey of Doctors Finds: Patient Requests Denied: 5% Admit Giving Injections—More Say They Would Do So If Procedure Were Legal." *New York Times*, April 23.

———. 1998c. "Guide Covers Territory Suicide Law Does Not Explore." *New York Times*, April 21.

———. 1998d. "In Death, the Goal Is No Questions Asked." *New York Times*, April 26.

———. 1998e. "Study Finds Pain of Oldest Is Ignored in Nursing Homes." *New York Times*, June 17.

Stone, Jim. 1994. "Advance Directives, Autonomy and Unintended Death." *Bioethics* 8(3): 223–46.

Stone, Julie. 1994. "Withholding Life-Sustaining Treatment: the Ultimate Decision." *New Law Journal* 144(6635): 205–206.

Stout, David. 1997. "From Emotional to Intellectual, Secular to Religious." *The New York Times*, June 27.

Stryker, Jeff. 1996. "Right to Die: Life After Quinlan." *New York Times*, March 31.

Sudnow, David. 1967. *Passing On: The Social Organization of Dying*. Englewood Cliffs, N.J.: Prentice-Hall.

Sutherland, John. 1992. "How to Die." *London Review of Books*, February 13.

Tallis, Raymond. 1996. "Is There a Slippery Slope?—Arguments for and against the Various Definitions of Euthanasia." *Medicine*, January 12.

Taylor, Sandra J. 1987. *In Everything There Is a Season: A Discussion of Euthanasia*. Kingston: Queen's University.

———. 1995. *Empathy, Care, and End of Life Decisions*. Kingston: Queen's University.

Teengel, Erwin. 1964. *Suicide and Attempted Suicide*. New York: Penguin Books.

Termination of Life by a Doctor in the Netherlands, The. 1995. Ministry of Foreign Affairs, Ministry of Justice, Ministry of Health, Welfare and Sport, the Hague.

Thorton, James, and Earl Winkler, eds. 1988. *Ethics and Aging*. Vancouver: University of British Columbia Press.

Tilden, V., S. Tolle, M. Lee, and C. Nelson. 1996. "Oregon's Physician-Assisted Suicide Vote: Its Effect on Palliative Care." *Nursing Outlook* 44(2): 80–83.

Tolchin, Martin. 1989. "When Long Life Is Too Much: Suicide Rises Among Elderly." *New York Times*, July 19.

Tomlinson T., K. Howe, M. Notman, and D. Rossmiller. 1990. "An Empirical Study of Proxy Consent for Elderly Persons." *Gerontologist* 30(1): 54–64.

Toulmin, Stephen. 1989. "How Medicine Saved the Life of Ethics." In *Contemporary Issues in Bioethics*. Eds. Tom L. Beauchamp and LeRoy Walters. Belmont, Calif.: Wadsworth.

Tribe, D., and G. Korgaonkar. 1993. "Withdrawal of Medical Treatment." *Journal of the Medical Defense Union* 2: 42–44.

Tronto, Joan C. 1993. *Moral Boundaries: A Political Argument for an Ethic of Care*. New York: Routledge.

Urofsky, Melvin I. 1993. *Letting Go: Death, Dying and the Law*. New York: Charles Scribners Sons.

Van Biema, David. 1997. "Fatal Doses: Assisted Suicide Soars in an Afflicted Community." *Time* (February 17): 53.

van Delden, Johannes J. M., et al. 1993. "The Remmelink Study: Two Years Later." *Hastings Center Report* 23(6): 24–32.

van der Burg, Wibren. 1992. "The Slippery-Slope Argument." *Journal of Clinical Ethics* 3(4): 256–69.

Van Hoof, Anton. 1960. *From Autothanasia to Suicide: Self Killing in Classical Antiquity*. London: Routledge.

Veatch, Robert M. 1989a. *Death, Dying and the Biological Revolution: Our Last Quest for Responsibility*. New Haven, Conn., and London: Yale University Press.

———, ed. 1989b. *Medical Ethics*. Boston: Jones and Bartlett.

Verhovek, Sam Howe. 1998. "Legal Suicide Has Killed 8, Oregon Says: A Report that Offers a Stark Glimpse into Legally Assisted Suicide." *New York Times*, August 19.

Vesey, Godrey, and Paul Foulkes. 1990. *Collins Dictionary of Philosophy*. London: Collins.

Vezeau, Toni M. 1992. "Caring: From Philosophical Concerns to Practice." *Journal of Clinical Ethics* 3(1): 18–21.

Voigt, Robert. 1995. "Euthanasia and HIV Disease: How Can Physicians Respond?" *Journal of Palliative Care* 11(2): 38–41.

Volicer, Ladislav. 1986. "Need for Hospice Approach to Treatment of Patients with Advanced Progressive Dementia." *Journal of the American Geriatrics Society* 34(9): 655–58.

Vries, B., S. Bluck, and J. Birren. 1993. "The Understanding of Death and Dying in a Life-Span Perspective." *Gerontologist* 33(3): 366–72.

Wal, G., and R. Dillman. 1994. "Euthanasia in the Netherlands." *British Medical Journal* 308: 1346–49.

Walker, R., R. Schonwetter, D. Kramer, and B. Robinson. 1995. "Living Wills and Resuscitation Preferences in an Elderly Population." *Archives of Internal Medicine* 155: 171–75.

Walton, Douglas N. 1979. *On Defining Death: An Analytic Study of the Concept of Death in Philosophy and Medical Ethics.* Montreal: McGill-Queen's University Press.

Wanzer, S., D. Federman, et al. 1989. "The Physician's Responsibility Towards Hopelessly Ill Patients—A Second Look." *New England Journal of Medicine* 320: 844–49.

Ward, B., and P. Tate. 1994. "Attitudes Among NHS Doctors to Requests for Euthanasia." *British Medical Journal* 308: 1332–34.

Wass, Hannalore, Felix Berardo, and Robert Neimeyer, eds. 1987. *Dying: Facing the Facts*, 2d ed. New York: Hemisphere.

Watts, D., and T. Howell. 1992. "Assisted Suicide Is Not Voluntary Active Euthanasia." *Journal of the American Geriatrics Society* 40(10): 1043–46.

Webb, Marilyn. 1998. "At the End of Life, A Blind Bureaucracy." *New York Times,* March 11.

Webber, P., P. Fox, and D. Burnette. 1994. "Living Alone with Alzheimer's Disease: Effects on Health and Social Service Utilization Patterns." *Gerontologist* 34(1): 8–14.

Weber, Arnott. 1997. "A Kinder, Gentler Way to Suicide." *Globe and Mail,* October 18.

Weiler, Ken. 1991. "Substitute Decision Makers in Health Care Treatment Decisions." *Journal of Professional Nursing* 7(5): 268.

Weinstein, Michael M. 1998. "Patient's Rights: Getting Litigious with H.M.O.'s: Three Studies Say the Legal System Fails Injured Patients." *New York Times,* July 19.

Weir, Robert F. 1992. "The Morality of Physician-Assisted Suicide." *Law, Medicine and Health Care* 20(1–2): 116–26.

———. 1997. *Physician-Assisted Suicide.* Bloomington: Indiana University Press.

Weisman, Avery. 1972. *On Dying and Denying.* New York: Behavioral Publications.

———. 1993. *The Vulnerable Self: Confronting The Ultimate Questions.* New York: Insight Books.

Wells, C. 1994. "Patients, Consent and Criminal Law." *Journal of Social Welfare and Family Law* 1: 65–78.

Wennberg, Robert N. 1989. *Terminal Choices: Euthanasia, Suicide, and the Right to Die*. Grand Rapids, Mich.: Eerdman's.

Whytehead, Lawrence, and Paul Chidwick, eds. 1980. *Dying: Considerations Concerning the Passage from Life to Death*. Toronto: Anglican Book Centre.

Wilkes, Paul. 1996. "The Next Pro-Lifers." *New York Times Magazine*, July 21.

———. 1997. "Dying Well Is the Best Revenge." *New York Times Magazine*, July 6.

Williams, Glanville. 1981. "Euthanasia Legislation: A Rejoinder to the Nonreligious Objections." In *Biomedical Ethics*. 3d ed. Eds. Thomas A. Mappes and Jane S. Zembaty. New York: McGraw-Hill.

Wilson, Deborah. 1993. "Rodriguez's Final Question: Who Owns My Life?" *Globe and Mail*, May 20.

Wilson, E. O. 1978. *On Human Nature*. Cambridge, Mass.: Harvard University Press.

Wrenn, K., and S. Brody. 1992. "Do-Not-Resuscitate Orders in the Emergency Department." *American Journal of Medicine* 92: 129–33.

WuDunn, Sheryl. 1997. "The Face of the Future in Japan: Economic Threat of Aging Populace." *New York Times*, September 2.

Young, E., and S. Jex. 1992. "The Patient Self-Determination Act: Potential Ethical Quandries and Benefits." *Cambridge Quarterly of Healthcare Ethics* 2: 107–15.

Zweibel, N., and C. Cassel. 1989. "Treatment Choices at the End of Life: A Comparison of Decisions by Older Patients and Their Physician-Selected Proxies." *Gerontologist* 29(5): 615–21.

MEDIA SECTION

The following are newspaper, magazine, and television items that appeared without authorial attribution. They are listed in reverse chronological order. In gathering and using media items, we relied most heavily on the *New York Times* because of its coverage, circulation, and general reputation, but also to provide an impression of the amount of coverage given to the issue of assisted suicide by one major U.S. national newspaper. We also found that many articles on the topic carried by other newspapers were attributed to the *New York Times*. The Canadian press is represented mostly by the *Globe and Mail* for similar reasons.

"Judge Orders Kevorkian To Be Tried For Murder." *New York Times*, December 10, 1998.

"Virginia's Top Court Rejects Appeal in Right-to-Die Case." *New York Times*, October 3, 1998.

"Family Will Allow a Comatose Man to Die." *New York Times*, September 29, 1998.

"Overreaching on Assisted Suicide." *New York Times*, September 17, 1998.

"Michigan to Decide on Doctor-Aided Suicide." *New York Times*, July 22, 1998.

"Michigan Demands Kevorkian Records." (Kingston, Ontario) *Whig-Standard*, July 18, 1998.

"Ban on Assisted Suicide." *New York Times*, July 4, 1998.

"Assisted Suicide, at State Discretion." *New York Times*, June 8, 1998.

"Kevorkian Offers Organs In Assisted-Suicide Case." *New York Times*, June 8, 1998.

"A Better Death in Oregon." *New York Times*, March 28, 1998.

"Hospital Worker Admits Killing Up to 50 Patients, Official Says." *New York Times*, March 28, 1998.

"Kevorkian Delivers Another Body to Hospital." *New York Times*, March 28, 1998.

"Quebec Fighting High Suicide Rate: Government Sets Aside Additional $700,000 for Prevention Programs, Public Education." *Globe and Mail*, February 3, 1998.

"Justice Dept. Bars Punishing Oregon Doctor Aiding Suicides." *New York Times*, January 24, 1998.

"Latimer's sentence on trial (II)." *Globe and Mail*, December 2, 1997.

"Latimer's sentence on trial (I)." *Globe and Mail*, December 2, 1997.

"Why Latimer was sentenced to only two years." *Globe and Mail*, December 2, 1997.

"Parliament and Assisted Suicide." *Globe and Mail*, November 8, 1997.

"Kevorkian Lawyer Cited in Note on Body." *New York Times*, October 15, 1997.

"H.M.O.'s Seen as Easing Death for the Elderly." *New York Times*, September 24, 1997.

"Kevorkian in New Suicide." *New York Times*, September 22, 1997.

"Kevorkian Is Called Irresponsible for Role in Woman's Suicide." *New York Times*, September 9, 1997.

"Florida High Court Upholds State Ban on Assisted Suicide." *New York Times*, July 18, 1997.

"Two Days that Shaped the Law." *New York Times*, June 28, 1997. (Editorial on four key Supreme Court decisions, including the assisted-suicide decision. Stresses continuing debate on the issue.)

"Woman's Kin Hires Kevorkian Lawyer." *New York Times*, June 28, 1997.

"Doctors Design Rules On Care for the Dying." *New York Times*, June 23, 1997

"Mistrial Declared in Kevorkian Case After Lawyer's Statement," *New York Times*, June 13, 1997.

"Kevorkian Trial: Jury Selection Begins." *USA Today*, June 9, 1997.

"It's Young vs. Old in Germany as the Welfare State Fades." *New York Times*, June 4, 1997.

"Health and the Aged." *Globe and Mail*, May 10, 1997.

"Kevorkian Lawyer Tied to Suicide in Michigan." *New York Times*, April 10, 1997.

"Stop Aid, State Tells Kevorkian." *New York Times*, April 5, 1997.

"Australia Strikes Down a State Suicide Law." *New York Times*, March 25, 1997.

"Congress Weighs More Regulation on Managed Care." *New York Times*, March 10, 1997.

"Kevorkian Lawyer Gives Rationale for a Suicide." *New York Times*, March 8, 1997.

"Suicide Law Withstands a Challenge." *New York Times*, Febuary 28, 1997. (Oregon law upheld.)

"Kevorkian Is Silent on 2 More Deaths." *New York Times*, Febuary 4, 1997.

"Assisted Suicide and the Law." *New York Times*, January 6, 1997.

"Court Denies Kevorkian Has a Right to Aid Suicide." *New York Times*, January 6, 1997.

"Before the Court, the Sanctity of Life and Death." *New York Times*, January 5, 1997. (Includes disturbing comparative photographs of Mary Bowen Hall.)

"Missouri Drops an Assisted-Suicide Case." *New York Times*, December 27, 1996.

"Clinton Administration Asks Supreme Court to Rule Against Assisted Suicide: Contrasting Life Support Withheld and Death Brought About." *New York Times*, November 13, 1996.

"Another Body Left at Hospital by Kevorkian." *New York Times*, October 18, 1996.

"Till Death Do Us Part," *Dateline*, NBC, September 27, 1996 (Program on George Delury's assisting the suicide of his wife, Myrna Lebov, on July 4, 1995).

"Australian Man First in World to Die With Legal Euthanasia." *New York Times*, September 26, 1996.

"Clash in Detroit." *New York Times*, Aug. 20, 1996.

"Question of Family Violence Arises in a Kevorkian Suicide Case," *New York Times*, August, 18, 1996.

"A.M.A. Keeps Its Policy Against Aiding Suicide," *New York Times*, June 26, 1996.

"Doctor Charged In Man's Suicide: AIDS Specialist Prescribed Pills." *Globe and Mail*, June 21, 1996.

"Kevorkian Assists Woman from New Jersey in Dying." *New York Times*, June 12, 1996.

"Man Ordered to Live with Wife Who Had Consulted Kevorkian." *New York Times*, June, 12, 1996.

"Man Who Helped Wife Die to Serve 6 Months." *New York Times*, May 18, 1996.

"Jury Acquits Kevorkian in Common-Law Case; 'This Will Be the Last Kevorkian Trial,' a Lawyer Says." *New York Times*, May 15, 1996.

"The Kevorkian Verdict," *Frontline*, WBGH (Boston) Educational Foundation, aired on Public Broadcasting System, May 14, 1996. (Includes interviews with Drs. Arthur Caplan and Timothy Quill, as well as courtroom coverage and film of Dr. Kevorkian and individuals he assisted in committing suicide.) Transcripts are available from PBS.

"Dr. Kevorkian on Trial, with Hints of the Future." *New York Times*, May 14, 1996.

"Kevorkian Back at Trial as Talk of Detroit Is of Another Suicide." *New York Times*, May 10, 1996.

"Bastable Tried to 'Wake Up Parliament': Assisted Suicide Hastened by Chrétien Snub of Meeting Attempt, Right to Die Society Says." *Globe and Mail*, May 9, 1996.

"Doctor Death Ignores Legalities on Mission of Mercy." *Globe and Mail*, May 9, 1996.

"Tape Recalls a Canadian's Gratitude to Kevorkian." *New York Times*, May 9, 1996.

"Kevorkian Repeatedly Disrupts His Trial, Calling It a Lynching." *New York Times*, May 7, 1996.

"Appeals Set Back Kevorkian Trial Repeatedly." *New York Times*, May 5, 1996.

"Death at Your Fingertips." *Sydney Morning Herald*, April 17, 1996.

"Lining Up For Battle." *Sydney Morning Herald*, April 17, 1996.

"Press 'Yes' to Die: Why Jan Culhane Hopes to Choose Death by Computer." *Sydney Morning Herald*, April 17, 1996.

"The Justices' Life-or-Death Choices." *New York Times*, April 7, 1996.

"MDs Can Aid Suicides, U.S. Court Rules." *Globe and Mail*, April 3, 1996.

"The Right to Die." *Economist*, September 17, 1994.

"To Cease upon the Midnight." *Economist*, September 17, 1994.

"Dutch Soften Law on Euthanasia." *Globe and Mail*, February 10, 1993.

"Doctor Charged with Murder in Assisted Suicides." *Globe and Mail*, February 6, 1992.

"Suicide Rate for Men Jumps 42% in 20 Years." *Globe and Mail*, March 27, 1991.

"When the Choice Is to Die." *Globe and Mail*, July 24, 1989.

"Survivors." *Currents*, WNET-TV, Boston (channel 13, New York), September 25, 1988.

WORLD WIDE WEB

Links to hundreds of sites offering relevant material may be found on the Internet. (In mid-1996 one of us searched for the phrase "assisted suicide" as an initial test and found *forty thousand* relevant articles, of which the first four hundred were available for downloading.) *Yahoo* is a good place to start searching (http://www.yahoo.com). Other useful search engines are *Excite* (http://www.excite.com) and *Altavista* (http://www.altavista.digital.com). One of the sites available from *Yahoo* is *The Euthanasia World Directory on the World Wide Web*. Another interesting site is the *New York Times* forum, which includes discussion of assisted suicide (http://forums.nytimes.com). Also of interest for American articles: http://www.rights.org/~deathnet/USNews_current.html, and for Canadian and international articles: http://www.rights.org/~deathnet/wnews_current.html. Two other sites worthy of note are http://www.efn.org/~ergo/ (Pro-Choice), and http://www.euthanasia.com (Pro-Life). Note that Web addresses change fairly often but can usually be tracked down through the previously mentioned search engines.

INDEX